BOOKS AVAILABLE IN THE
LIVINGSTONE MEDICAL TEXT SERIES

The Author

C.B.S. SCHOFIELD

M.D., F.R.C.P.E. & G.
Consultant in Sexually Transmitted Diseases, Glasgow

Sexually Transmitted Diseases

C.B.S. SCHOFIELD

Second Edition

CHURCHILL LIVINGSTONE
EDINBURGH LONDON AND NEW YORK
1975

CHURCHILL LIVINGSTONE

Medical Division of Longman Group Limited

Distributed in the United States of America by Longman Inc., New York
and by associated companies, branches and representatives throughout the
world.

© Longman Group Limited 1972, 1975

First Edition 1972
Second Edition 1975

ISBN 0 443 01159 1

Printed in Great Britain

Computer Typesetting by Print Origination,
Bootle, Merseyside, L20 6NS

Preface

I am indebted to the reviewers of the first edition of this book for the many constructive criticisms made. These have been of great help in the preparation of this edition. Possibly not every point has been taken up, but they were all noted and I hope that at least the errors have been corrected.

Sexually transmitted diseases are the commonest communicable diseases found in the world today, and the numbers of patients treated for them continues to increase each year. The rise in incidence has taken place despite rapid advances in diagnostic facilities and the ready availability of specific drugs with which to cure them. Only a minority of these patients suffer from the venereal diseases, syphilis, gonorrhoea, chancroid, lymphogranuloma venereum and granuloma inguinale. The majority of patients suffer from conditions such as non-specific urethritis, trichomoniasis, genital candidosis, scabies, warts, molluscum contagiosum, phthirius, pubis infestation and herpes genitalis. In addition many patients have genital conditions, not sexually transmitted, which have to be differentiated from those which are. Because these diseases can affect anyone, the non-promiscuous as well as the promiscuous, and have such a wide variety of signs, symptoms and associated social complications, doctors and social workers in many fields of work are liable to have to deal with them. To do this properly, they need to understand the medico-social management which is required if these diseases are to be contained if not controlled.

A number of additions have had to be made to certain chapters to bring the material up to date, consequent upon the increase in interest in the sexually transmitted diseases shown by scientists in many of the fields of medicine over the past few years. The use of automated serological tests for syphilis has become much more widespread, specific serological tests for *Chlamydia* have been developed and one for gonorrhoea has been introduced. Immunopathological investigations have increased our knowledge of the humoral and cellular responses of the host to infection by *T. pallidum, N. gonorrhoeae* and the *Chlamydiae.*

In Glasgow we have noted changes in the social background of patients attending with gonorrhoea. They have become younger, especially the women; fewer are married, with increases in the number of men who are separated and of single women. Prostitutes are now only rarely named as the source of infection.

Once again, it is a great pleasure to be able to express my thanks and appreciation to all those who have helped in the revision of this book, particularly to Dr. T.F. Elias-Jones, Director of the City Laboratory, Glasgow, to Mr. Sidney Bindemann, Research Psychologist in the Glasgow Department of Sexually Transmitted Diseases and especially to my colleague Dr. George Masterton. I must also express my gratitude to the publishers for their continued support and consideration and last but not least, to my secretary, Mrs. Linda Smith.

C.B.S. SCHOFIELD

Contents

1. Anatomy of Genital Tracts, Rectum and Anus

The sexually transmitted diseases affect principally the reproductive organs and the urinary tract and, to a lesser extent, the anus and rectum. A knowledge of the relevant anatomy, histology and lymphatic drainage is necessary to appreciate the significance of clinical findings, to correlate those associated with one lesion or distinguish between those due to more than one condition.

MALE

Urethra

The urethra extends from the bladder neck to the external urethral meatus and is a potential canal, the walls being in contact except during micturition. This, together with its 'S' shaped course and length, 20 to 22 cm, makes the drainage of any urethral discharge difficult. Anatomically the urethra is divided into three parts: prostatic, membranous and penile, but clinically into only two: the posterior urethra which includes the prostatic and membranous parts, and the anterior urethra which corresponds to the penile urethra.

Prostatic urethra

The prostatic urethra descends vertically from the internal urethral orifice for about 3 cm through the prostate gland. At the level of the urogenital diaphragm it becomes the membranous urethra. Proximally the mucous membrane is continuous with the transitional epithelium of the bladder, and distally with the columnar epithelium of the membranous urethra, prostatic gland and ducts, and the common ejaculatory ducts. On the posterior wall is a narrow longitudinal ridge called the urethral crest or verumontanum. It is about 15 mm long and has on it an elevation, the colliculus seminalis, in the centre of which is the slit-like orifice of the prostatic utricle. On either side of this

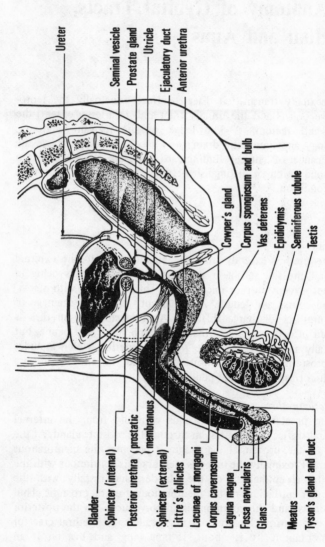

Fig. 1 Anatomical diagram of male genito-urinary tract (facing). (Reproduced from A. S. Grimble: *McLachlan's Handbook of Diagnosis and Treatment of Venereal Diseases*, 5th edn. Edinburgh: Livingstone.)

orifice lie the two small openings of the common ejaculatory ducts. Lateral to the urethral crest are shallow depressions, the prostatic sinuses, which receive the ducts of the lateral lobes of the prostate, those from the middle lobe opening above the crest.

The prostate gland is about the size and shape of a chestnut. Its apex lies on the urogenital diaphragm and posteriorly it is in contact with the anterior rectal wall. The prostate consists of three lobes, the two lateral ones which surround the urethra being separated posteriorly by a median groove, the middle one lying above and between the ejaculatory ducts. A thin fibro-muscular capsule encloses the glandular tissue which is of branched tubules, lined by columnar epithelium and whose ducts open into the prostatic urethra as do the common ejaculatory ducts which pass through the gland substance.

The testes and epididymes hang by the spermatic cords within the scrotal sac, the left lower than the right. The testis is an oval structure to which the epididymis is attached posterially. The anterior and lateral surfaces are covered by the visceral layer of the tunica vaginalis. The body of the testis is covered with fibrous tissue, the tunica albuginea, which is thicker beneath the epididymis. It forms the mediastinum testis which is pierced postero-superiorly by the seminiferous tubules, united into about 20 efferent ductules which form the upper pole or globus major of the epididymes. The testis is a lobulated gland, each lobule containing one to three convoluted tubules whose average length is about 1 metre. Each of these seminiferous tubules has a basement layer of connective tissue within which lie epithelial cells in three irregular layers. The outer layer is of cuboidal cells dividing to form a second layer of somewhat larger cells which are the precursors of the spermatozoa; these are liberated and set free into the lumen of the tubule. The epididymis is the first part of the efferent duct of the testis. This highly convoluted muscular tube, lined with ciliated columnar epithelium, is 5 to 6 metres long. It is divided into three parts from above down: the globus major, the body, and the globus minor or lower pole closely bound to the body of the testis leading to the vas deferens.

The vasa deferentia are continuations of the canals of the epididymes. They are thick-walled, muscular-coated tubes, about 40 cm long lined with non-ciliated columnar epithelium. Each vas starts at the lower pole of the epididymis, behind which it ascends, to become the most easily palpable part of the spermatic cord as it passes up to the external inguinal ring and into the inguinal canal. At the internal inguinal ring the vas leaves the blood vessels and nerves to pass downwards and backwards along the pelvic wall towards the medial aspect of the seminal vesicle. At this point it becomes sacculated forming the ampulla, before contracting to join the duct of the seminal vesicle and become the common ejaculatory duct.

The seminal vesicles are two coiled, sacculated tubes about 5 cm long which store seminal fluid. They are placed between the fundus of the bladder and the rectum, lying lateral to the vasa deferentia which they join at the base of the prostate. Each consists of a tube, coiled upon itself and giving off several irregular diverticula. The epithelium is columnar in type with goblet-cells present in the diverticula adding a secretion to the seminal fluid.

Membranous urethra

The membranous urethra is the shortest (1·5 cm), least dilatable and, with the exception of the external urinary meatus, the narrowest part of the urethra. It pierces the two fascial layers of the urogenital diaphragm in a curve downwards and forwards. Lined with columnar epithelium and surrounded by the compressor urethrae muscle, it is continuous with the prostatic urethra proximally and with the bulbous portion of the penile urethra distally with which its columnar epithelium is continuous.

Cowper's glands lie, one on each side, postero-laterally to the membranous urethra. Each is a firm, round and lobulated mass, the size of a pea but decreasing in size with age. The acini are lined with columnar epithelium as are the ducts, which run forward for about 3 cm before opening on the floor of the bulbous urethra.

Anterior urethra

The anterior urethra extends from the termination of the membranous urethra to the external meatus, and is about 15 cm long. It is embedded within the corpus spongiosum; the proximal portion, lying between the anterior layer of the urogenital diaphragm and the peno-scrotal junction, is termed the bulbous urethra. Dilated to a diameter of 2·5 cm it is fixed to the suspensory ligament of the penis. The distal portion, pendulous, distensile and mobile, is about 6 mm in diameter with a terminal dilation, the fossa navicularis. The external urethral meatus is bounded on either side by a small labium, upon which opens the para-urethral duct, a small blind channel which has run parallel to the terminal urethra. The anterior urethra is lined with columnar epithelium except for the fossa navicularis where it is stratified and squamous, continuous with that of the glans penis. The mucous membrane of the side walls and roof of the urethra is studded with the ducts of many Littré's glands which are simple, compound or racemose, lined with columnar epithelium and secreting mucus; those in the roof usually penetrate the mucous membrane within the lacunae of Morgani, blind recesses pointing forward. The largest of the lacunae is situated just proximal to the fossa navicularis and is termed the lacuna magna or valve of Guérin. Congenital defects of the urethra occur occasionally. The most common hypospadias, is a cleft in the floor of the urethra due to arrest of union in the mid-line. This occurs with varying degrees of severity, the urethra opening at the base of the glans, at the peno-scrotal junction or in the perineum and associated with a cleft scrotum. A much rarer condition, epispadias, occurs when there is an apparent deficiency of the roof of the urethra. This varies in extent, but when complete is associated with extroversion of the bladder.

Penis

In addition to the corpus spongiosum surrounding the urethra, there are two other masses of erectile tissue, the corpora cavernosa, within the penis. Anteriorly the corpus spongiosum suddenly expands to form an obtuse cone, the glans penis, which is normally covered by the prepuce. The projecting base of the glans is named the corona, and the constriction behind it the coronal sulcus. On the ventral surface of the glans is a small median fold, the fraenum, which extends from below the urethral orifice to the deep surface of the prepuce.

Tyson's glands lie just proximal to the coronal sulcus, into which their ducts open on either side of the fraenum. They secrete sebaceous material as do a number of smaller glands situated around the coronal sulcus. Each Tyson's gland consists of a cluster of oval alveoli with a polyhedral columnar lining, which continues into the duct. The cells within the lumen of the alveoli are filled with fat and when they disrupt form sebum.

The prepuce covers the glans penis, being separated by a potential space. The skin of the prepuce is very thin and dark, as is that of the penis, where it is loosely connected with the underlying fibrous envelope which binds the corpora. The under surface of the prepuce and the glans is covered with squamous epithelium, continuous with that of the urethral orifice. In some adults the free margin of the prepuce is too tight for it to be retracted over the glans (phimosis), or having been retracted it cannot be replaced over the corona of the glans (paraphimosis).

FEMALE

Vulva

The vulva, the female external genital organ, includes the mons pubis, the labia majora, the labia minora, the clitoris, the vestibule of the vagina, Bartholin's glands and the hymen.

The mons pubis is a prominence, overlying the symphysis pubis and formed by a subcutaneous pad of fat, which becomes covered with hair at puberty.

The labia majora, two prominent longitudinal masses of fat and areolar tissue, extend posteriorly from the mons pubis to meet at the posterior fourchette, between which and the anus is the gynaecological perineum, some 3 cm in length. They are the anatomical equivalent of the scrotum in the male. Externally in adults the skin is pigmented and covered with hair but the inner surfaces are smooth and studded with many sebaceous glands.

The labia minora are two small cutaneous folds lying between the labia majora. Anteriorly they form the prepuce of the clitoris, then extend postero-laterally to terminate on each side of the vaginal orifice. Their medial surfaces contain many sebaceous follicles.

The clitoris is an erectile structure, and like the penis has a body and a highly sensitive glans. It is situated at the apex of the vestibule, partially hidden between the anterior ends of the labia minora.

The vestibule is that area bounded by the labia minora and into which open the external urethral meatus, the vagina and the ducts of Bartholin's glands.

Bartholin's glands lie, one on either side, within the posterior third of each labium majus. They are racemose mucus-secreting glands lined with columnar epithelium, as is each duct, which

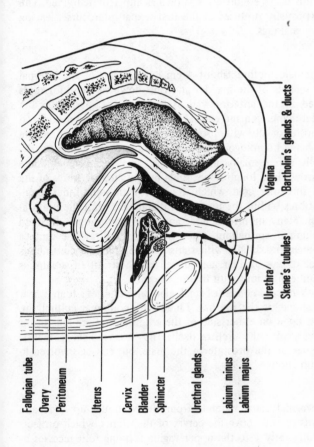

Fig. 2 Anatomical diagram of female genito-urinary tract (facing). (Reproduced from A. S. Grimble: *McLachlan's Handbook of Diagnosis and Treatment of Venereal Diseases*, 5th edn. Edinburgh: Livingstone.)

Fallopian tube
Ovary
Peritoneum

Uterus

Cervix
Bladder
Sphincter

Urethral glands

Labium minus
Labium majus

Vagina
Bartholin's glands & ducts

Urethra
Skene's tubules

extends about 2 cm to open lateral to the hymen, within a mucosal fold.

The hymen is a thin fold of mucous membrane at the vaginal orifice. Its free margin may vary in shape from a slit to a ring; it may be absent or form a complete septum across the vaginal orifice; this latter condition is known as imperforate hymen. The hymen is usually ruptured at the first sexual intercourse, leaving small hymenal tags.

Urethra

The female urethra, about 4 cm long, begins at the internal urethral meatus of the bladder and runs downward and forwards embedded in the anterior wall of the vagina. It perforates the urogenital diaphragm and ends at the external urethral meatus, an antero-posterior slit with prominent margins, 2·5 cm behind the clitoris, being homologous with the posterior urethra of the male. The walls are normally in apposition, the mucous membrane being thrown into longitudinal folds by the circular fibres of the external muscular coat which, together with some inner longitudinal fibres within the urogenital diaphragm form the urethral sphincter. Many minute lacunae and small urethral glands, lined with columnar epithelium, open into the urethra. The urethra itself is lined proximally with transitional epithelium continuous with that of the bladder, and distally with stratified squamous epithelium continuous with that of the vulva.

Skene's tubules consist of small glandular tubules situated near the lower end of the urethra. Lined with columnar epithelium, the ducts open on either side of the external urethral meatus, or occasionally into the urethra itself. They are vestigial remnants, homologues of the prostate in the male, but can be involved in genital infections.

Vagina

The vaginal canal extends from the vestibule upwards and backwards to end above the cervix of the uterus, which projects postero-inferiorly into the upper vagina forming four recesses or fornices. The posterior fornix lies behind and above the cervix and is much larger than the anterior and lateral ones. The vagina consists of an internal mucous membrane and a muscular coat separated by a layer of erectile tissue. The anterior wall measures about 8 cm and the posterior 12 cm, but the vagina can distend in length as well as breadth, especially posteriorly. The lower part is 'H' shaped in cross-section, with well-marked longitudinal folds and transverse ridges which are less well marked in the upper and wider part. The stratified squamous epithelium is devoid of glands and is kept moist by serous transudates. At birth the mucous membrane is of the adult type owing to the presence of maternal hormones, but soon becomes columnar and thin, with alkaline secretions until puberty. Then, under the control of oestrogens the cells become laden with glycogen. This is acted upon by lactobacilli, (Döderlein's bacilli), and the environment kept acid. On the withdrawal of oestrogens at the menopause the mucous membrane tends to become thin and atrophic, there is less glycogen in the cells and the pH rises to neutral.

Uterus

The uterus is a hollow, thick-walled, muscular, pear-shaped organ. The Fallopian tubes enter laterally into its upper part, whilst below its cavity communicates with the vagina. It is about 7·5 cm long and, in the upper part, 5 cm broad and 2·5 cm thick. It is divided into two parts at the isthmus, the body above and below the smaller part, the cervix.

The cervix is about 2·5 cm long and is cylindrical in shape. Its external os has an anterior and posterior lip; in the nullipara the os may be circular but appears as a transverse slit in parous women. The canal is fusiform, its surface ridged in a branching fashion. Many racemose glands, lined with columnar epithelium open into the canal which has ciliated columnar epithelium in the upper two-thirds below which it loses its cilia, while close to the external os it is lined with stratified squamous epithelium continuous with that of the vagina.

The body of the uterus when normally anteverted on the cervix rests on the bladder. It is suspended from the walls of the pelvis by the broad ligaments, two peritoneal folds which form a septum across the female pelvis. The mucous membrane lining the uterus (the endometrium) is thick and its free surface consists of ciliated columnar epithelium continuous with that of the upper cervical canal and the Fallopian tubes.

The Fallopian tubes and ovaries

The Fallopian tubes are about 10 cm long and lie in the upper margins of the broad ligaments. The medial openings into the upper uterine cavity are very narrow indeed while the lateral openings into the peritoneal cavity, close to the ovary, are wide and lie at the base of a trumpet-shaped expansion, the infundibulum. From the free margin of the infundibulum extend a number of fimbriae, one of which is attached to the ovary.

The ovaries are oval-shaped organs homologous with the testes in the male. Each is attached to the back of the broad ligament and, by the round ligament, to the uterus. It lies behind and below the Fallopian tube, one of the fimbriae of which is attached to its lateral pole.

The anal canal and rectum

In men and women the anal canal extends 2 to 3 cm from the anus upwards and forwards, in males to the level of the apex of the prostate. It is usually only a potential canal, the lateral walls being in apposition. It has two sphincters, an external and internal, separated by the levatores ani. The peri-anal skin is thrown into a series of folds which converge on the orifice and are continued up the lower half of the canal to the junction of skin and mucous membrane which is indicated by an irregular white line. The upper half is lined with columnar epithelium, the mucous membrane being in vertical folds, the rectal columns, the infoldings of which join together to form crescentic valve like folds, the anal valves. The rectum, 12 cm long, extends from the anal canal to the level of the third sacral vertebra, taking an 'S' shaped course, the upper curve with its convexity to the back. The dilated lower part forms the ampulla, and when this is contracted the mucous membrane lies in longitudinal folds. There are at least three transverse semilunar folds; the valves of Houston, two on the right hand wall and one on the left. When the bowel is empty they overlap, often very tightly. The mucous membrane is columnar in type, with numerous glands lined by short columnar epithelium, the majority of the cells being goblet cells. Sub-epithelial solitary lymph nodules are also present in small numbers.

LYMPHATIC DRAINAGE

Of all the lymph glands which drain the genitalia, the rectum and the anus, only the inguinal glands are readily palpable. The lymph vessels and glands are to be found in relation to the blood vessels. The inguinal groups of glands drain via the external iliac group, through the common iliacs to the pre- or lateral aortic groups. The internal iliac group drain into the common iliac group while the sacral groups drain either into the internal or common iliac groups.

The genitalia

Males. The testis and epididymis drain directly to the lateral and pre-aortic lymph glands; the vas deferens to the external iliacs and the seminal vesicle to the internal and external iliac groups. The prostate drains chiefly to the sacral and internal iliac lymph glands, but some vessels go to the external iliac group. The prostatic and membranous urethra drain into the internal iliacs, but a few vessels may go to the external iliacs. The vessels of the anterior urethra and glans penis pass mainly to the deep inguinal lymph glands, but some may reach the superficial group while others go to the external iliacs. The skin of the external genitalia and perineum all drain into the superficial inguinal lymph glands.

Females. The ovary, like the testis, drains directly to the lateral and pre-aortic lymph glands. The Fallopian tubes and the body of the uterus drain mainly into the lateral and pre-aortic groups, but some vessels pass to the internal iliacs, and a few from the area of insertion of the tube into the uterus to the superficial inguinal group. Drainage from the cervix is in three directions: laterally to the external iliacs, postero-laterally to the internal iliacs and backwards to the sacral glands. The lymph vessels of the vagina anastomose with those of the cervix, rectum and vulva. The upper and middle vagina drains mainly into the external iliac lymph glands, while that part below the hymen drains into the superficial inguinal group, together with the vessels from the vulva and skin of the external genitalia and perineum.

The anal canal and rectum

The lymph vessels from the anus pass to the superficial inguinal lymph glands, those from the anal canal and lower rectum drain into the internal iliac glands. Vessels from the upper rectum initially traverse the pararectal group of lymph glands and then pass mainly to those at the bifurcation of the common iliac artery, but some from the highest pararectal lymph glands pass via glands in the pelvic mesocolon to the pre-aortic group around the origin of the inferior mesenteric artery.

FURTHER READING

Cunningham's Textbook of Anatomy (1943). 8th edn. Edited by J. C. Brash & E. B. Jamieson. London: Oxford Medical Publications.

Gray's Anatomy (1958). 32nd edn. Edited by T. B. Johnston, D. V. Davies & F. Davies. London: Longmans.

2. History Taking and Examination

HISTORY TAKING

The importance of obtaining an accurate case history is accepted in all fields of medicine, but can be vital in the sexually transmitted diseases as it saves so much time in arriving at an accurate diagnosis. When a patient attends a 'special clinic', he, or she, has suspected or accepted the possibility of such a disease, but elsewhere this is not necessarily so. Both the doctor and patient may be unaware of the nature of the disease initially and when the patient does realize it, guilt, remorse and fear may make him confused or recticent to admit to any form of sexual indiscretion. At this point, reassurance is needed that everything said will be treated in confidence. The young, single or unmarried can afford to be, and generally are, more forthright in these matters than the married, middle-aged or homosexual. Usually certain clues are available: symptoms often refer to the genitalia, but may be urinary or gynaecological, and follow either periods away from home at work, on business or holiday, after marital troubles or late night parties and too much to drink.

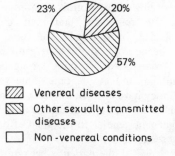

Fig. 3 Conditions treated in special clinics.

Good history taking is an art which rarely comes naturally but the techniques of interviewing are improved with practice and experience. Unfortunately the obvious and simple points too often appear to be neglected or have been forgotten by many doctors. The interview should take place in privacy, and it is essential to attain a rapport with every patient, no matter what or who he is. Every patient needs to feel that he is being heard with sympathy and without any apparent disapproval, so that the attitude of the doctor is all important.

Always let the patient tell his story in his own way, it saves time later. Note all the salient points, evasions, omissions and suspected inaccuracies, if necessary later clarifying the points by questioning, but never try to force the patient to admit to a lie; rather give him the opportunity to 'remember' correctly; otherwise, to save face, he may have to maintain the lie. The correct phrasing of questions is of the utmost importance; the use of leading questions may result in the patient giving the answers he thinks are wanted, whether true or not. A number of patients are semi-literate and have only a limited vocabulary, so use only those words they can comprehend. The majority of mistakes blamed on patients occur when there is a misunderstanding between doctor and patient, simple lack of communication. If a homosexual with urethral gonorrhoea is asked when he last had sex with a woman, he may honestly deny any such risk, and the doctor call him a liar, when in fact it was the question which was wrong. The initial question should have been worded to find out the occasions when the patient had sexual intercourse that could have resulted in infection, and subsequent ones to find out with whom. Correct wording of questions is most important.

One must always remember that men and women have different psychological backgrounds. Men tend to fear loss of potency and to be neurotic about their genitalia; many worry about nothing. Women fear anything wrong being discovered about their genitalia, and at the same time worry about the possible effect it may have on their unborn children. This appears to be more than modesty alone, as can be noted from the poor response by women in general to the great efforts made by the cervical cytology services.

Previous knowledge of the patient's background is usually of great value, but on occasions it can be misleading and one must never take on trust what one thinks one knows about a patient, for better or for worse. The results of careful clinical examination and of the laboratory findings are the only basis for a correct diagnosis, and if the patient's history does not agree with them, then it must be reviewed.

The case history, which should be entered in the patient's case notes at the time of interview, should contain the following information:

Demographic information. If not already known this should include age; sex; marital status (single, married and if separated, divorced or widowed and for how long); whether living at home, or if not, with whom; occupation, whether local or peripatetic, or if unemployed for how long and the reason; the patient's address and whether a resident or in transit; the country of birth and colour of skin.

The patient's complaints. It is important to know the duration, severity and course of all the symptoms; what treatment, if any, has been taken and with what results. It is a great help if the patient brings a sample of the drugs.

Exposure to infection. Note the dates or periods during which exposures to infection occurred, separating the marital or regular consort from all others, during the past three months or longer if necessary, and whether the association was hetero- or homosexual. Note also where the various exposures took place: locally, in the same country, or if abroad in which country.

Past history. Inquire about any previous sexually transmitted, genito-urinary or gynaecological conditions and their treatment, the results and any treatment reactions. Ask specifically about any possible penicillin reactions or a history of allergy.

Family history. When relevant, inquire about the health of parents and the cause of death; the birth order of siblings, the position of the patient in the family, and the health or causes of deaths of the siblings.

Female patients. A menstrual history should record any recent changes in the cycle and what contraceptives, if any, have been used in the past as well as the present. The pregnancy history should include the number of living children and their health, the causes of death of any who have died, and the dates of any miscarriages, abortions or still-births.

THE EXAMINATION

An examination is carried out not only to inspect and define the anatomical lesions but mainly to enable the appropriate specimens to be taken, upon which the correct laboratory tests can be carried out to make the diagnosis. The diagnosis of sexually transmitted diseases usually depends on either identifying the causal organism or detecting antibodies against them, both laboratory procedures. Microscopy can be carried out by any clinician but suitable microscopes are expensive; they do have some advantage that the diagnosis can be made immediately, whereas there may be a delay of up to a week in getting reports back from a laboratory. A microscope to carry out the routine investigations that are considered necessary should have a substage with Abbé, darkfield and phase contrast condensers, together with the appropriate objective lenses giving a magnification of X 1000, as the Wild M 20 microscope does. Many specialists also use a fluorescent microscope, such as the Gillett and Sibert Conference I.Q. Fluorescence Microscope which, with an ultra-violet light source and darkfield condenser, can identify *Neisseria gonorrhoeae* and TRIC agents *(Chlamydia)* using specific immunofluorescent stains. In every case when the clinician has made a diagnosis on the basis of his own laboratory findings he should ensure that they are confirmed by culture or serology carried out by the appropriate laboratories.

Genital examination

It is most important to establish and maintain a routine of genital examination, so that every patient is examined in the same careful and systematic manner, not only for the lesion complained of, but also that other lesions may be found that had not been mentioned, or noticed, by the patient; it is not uncommon for a patient to be suffering from more than one sexually transmitted disease at the same time. From the patient's point of view it is reassuring to see the doctor wash his hands with soap and water after, if not before, the examination and use a fresh pair of disposable or a clean pair of rubber gloves. It is worth remembering that patients do prefer to be examined by hands that are not only clean, but warm too.

Men

Patients should always be examined in a good light, and in daylight if possible, either standing up or lying on a couch. Initially they should at least be stripped from chest to knees. The skin of the trunk and thighs is examined for spots, rashes or burrows and scratch marks. In the latter case a scraping placed on a glass slide and treated with liquor potasseae should reveal the *Sarcoptes scabiei* or the eggs when viewed under low power of the microscope. The hair from pubis to anus is examined for *Phthirius pubis* or the nits. Palpate the inguinal fold for adenitis. If the glands are discrete, painless and rubbery and there is no other clinical evidence of contagious syphilis, a gland puncture may be necessary. After infiltrating the skin over the gland with 2 per cent procaine hydrochloride, an intramuscular needle, attached to a syringe containing 0·2 ml of normal saline, is inserted into the cortex, the gland being held steady, and the saline injected. The needle is moved around within the gland and the fluid aspirated, two drops at a time are placed on glass slides with a drop of normal saline as a diluent, if necessary, cover slips added and gently pressed together between pieces of filter paper. These wet films are examined for *Treponema pallidum* under a microscope with a darkground condenser. If there is a bubo or even sinuses, it may be necessary to aspirate some of the pus from which smears are made, fixed in methyl alcohol and later stained by Giemsa's method for Halberstaedter-Prowazek inclusions or sent to a laboratory in Hanks' medium or in sucrose potassium glutamate (S.P.G.) solution as soon as possible in an attempt to culture on BHK21 or Hela cells, *Chlamydia,* the causal organisms of lymphogranuloma venereum. Palpate the testes for swellings and tenderness or atrophy, the epididymes for scars, cysts or inflammation with swelling, tenderness and lateral rotation, and the vasa for funiculitis, with thickening and acute tenderness. Examine the skin of the scrotum and penis for nodular burrows and scratch marks, warts, rashes, erosions or ulcers. If contagious syphilis is suspected, and it should be in the case of all genital sores until proven otherwise, the lesion or lesions should be cleansed with a firm saline swab, abraided if necessary with the swab or a scarifier to obtain serum, from which several wet films are prepared as with the material obtained by gland puncture, and examined by darkground microscopy for *T. pallidum*. Scrapings from crops of erosions or vesicles are dropped into bijou bottles containing Hanks' Transport Medium for later culture for herpes simplex virus. Palpate the penis for peri-urethral and median raphe abscesses. If there is any pus available take specimens for stained smears and cultures. For smears, having cleaned the skin with a swab, use a sterile platinum loop and spread the material thinly on a glass slide, fix it by heat and stain it by Gram's method for microscopic diagnosis of *N. gonorrhoeae* and *Candida albicans*. For culture use a sterile charcoal impregnated swab to obtain the material which is then plunged deep into Stuart's Transport Medium for later culture in a laboratory of *N. gonorrhoeae, Trichomonas vaginalis* and *C. albicans*. A bottle of Transgrow nutritive transport medium can also be inoculated for culture of *N. gonorrhoeae,* but direct plating for culture can only be done by those who have an incubator on the premises. Material on a platinum loop is used to inoculate a plate of McLeod's chocolate agar or Thayer and Martin's medium for *N. gonorrhoeae,* Feinberg-Whittington or cysteine–peptone–liver–mallose (C.P.L.M.) mediums for *T. vaginalis* and Sabouraud's medium for *C. albicans*. If the patient is uncircumcised, retract the prepuce. If a phimosis prevents this, palpate through the prepuce for any mass and to elicit any sub-preputial discharge. With a fine rubber tube attached to a 10 ml syringe irrigate the sub-preputial sac with normal saline and prepare wet films for darkground examination of *T. pallidum, Vincent's* organisms and *T. vaginalis,* smears for staining for *N. gonorrhoeae* and *C. albicans* and cultures. In the circumcised, and when the prepuce can be retracted, examine the under-surface of the prepuce, glans penis, coronal sulcus and Tyson's glands for inflammation, erosions, ulcers, warts and a discharge or trauma to the fraenum. Make wet films for darkground examination as before but, if there is no evidence of syphilis and trichomoniasis is suspected, phase contrast microscopy can be used. This method is cleaner than the darkground method as oil is not needed between the slide and the sub-stage condenser, a great advantage when many slides have to be examined in a clinic. Take a smear for Gram staining and a specimen for culture. The urethral meatus and para-urethral ducts are examined for inflammation and a discharge: if present, the area is cleaned with a swab, smears taken for Gram staining for *N. gonorrhoeae* and *C. albicans,* a wet film for *T. vaginalis* and a specimen for culture of all three. It may be necessary to milk the terminal urethra forward to obtain a specimen of the discharge. The patient should now be asked to void urine into two glass or plastic urine jars, the two glass urine test, about 5 cm into the first one and the rest into the second, noting the quality of the stream. Some patients need a drink of water and others privacy before they can urinate. The specimen in each glass is examined for clarity or for haze due to pyuria, always remembering that phosphate crystals can make an alkaline urine hazy, the haze disappearing when the urine is made acid by adding a few drops of dilute acetic acid; for threads or specks in the urine, those due to pus sinking quickly, those of epithelium more slowly while mucus floats. It may be necessary to centrifuge a portion and examine the deposit by microscopy for leucocytes, red blood cells and organisms and by culture. The urine should next be screened for the presence of protein and sugar. Deep urethral scrapings, used for the diagnosis of chlamydial infections, are taken after micturition, the material being either spread thinly on to glass slides and fixed either in methyl alcohol for later identification of inclusion bodies or in acetone for 2 to 5 minutes for later fluorescent microscopy, or sent in Hank's medium for culture.

With the patient lying in the left or right lateral position and knees drawn well up, or standing with legs well apart and leaning over a couch the anus and peri-anal skin is examined for possible inflammation, discharge, erosions, ulcers and warts and from which the appropriate specimens are taken. Only Thayer and Martin's medium should be used for culture of *N. gonorrhoeae,* as it alone contains antibiotics which will kill off contiminating bowel organisms. If any abnormality is found, or if the patient is an admitted homosexual, confirmatory evidence such as funneling of the orifice with a lax anal sphincter and possibly a sentinal pile, may be noted, and the rectum examined by means of a proctoscope, searching for areas of induration, pus, erosions or ulcers and taking the necessary specimens. Digital rectal examination is needed to palpate the seminal vesicles, prostate and Cowper's glands but is deferred for a few days if the patient has a urethritis, by which time it will have responded to treatment. The seminal vesicles are not normally palpable, but when inflamed are swollen and tender as is the prostate, gentle palpation of which should produce sufficient secretions which, if milked along the length of the urethra, will produce a bead at the urethral orifice; from this bead are prepared a smear, wet films for microscopy, and material for culture. When swollen and inflamed, Cowper's glands can be palpated antero-laterally to the external rectal sphincter.

Women

The patient should be placed in the lithotomy position for

examination, and once again in a good light. Examination of the skin and inguinal folds is as for men, but in addition all lower abdominal scars should be noted as well as any excoriation of the perineum and inner thighs, the latter often caused by trichomoniasis. Examine the perineum, vulva, labia majora and minora for any discharge, inflammation, oedema, erosions, ulcers, warts, spots or rashes; clean by swabbing and take specimens for the appropriate tests. Separate the labia and palpate Bartholin's glands, noting any discharge from the ducts, swab clean the urethral orifice and Skene's tubules, milk the urethra and look for any discharges or inflammation. Take specimens for smears and cultures for *N. gonorrhoeae, T. vaginalis* and *C. albicans*. An immediate diagnosis of gonorrhoea is as important in women as in men, but Gram-stained smears do not reveal *N. gonorrhoeae* in women as easily as cultures, or as smears do in men, whereas staining by the rather more time consuming immunofluorescent method does. For this reason, in all new cases, duplicate smears are taken for each of those to be stained by Gram's method, and if the Gram-stained ones fail to reveal expected *N. gonorrhoeae,* the duplicates can then be used for fluorescent staining. Note also any erosions or ulcers and take specimens as required. Unless the patient is *virgo intacta* examine the vagina and cervix, using a bi-valve speculum of the appropriate size, the light being so directed as to give good illumination. Examine the vaginal walls for patches of inflammation and cheesy plaques of candidosis or more severe inflammation also affecting the cervix and associated with a frothy vaginal discharge due to trichomoniasis, *T. vaginalis* being most commonly isolated from secretions obtained from the posterior fornix. The cervix should be examined for cervicitis and erosions, which if indurated may be syphilitic and reveal *T. pallidum* from scrapings examined by darkground microscopy, or if inflammatory *N. gonorrhoeae* found by microscopy and culture. When there is a follicular cervicitis scrapings should be taken looking for *Chlamydia.* In those cases of *virgo intacta* it may be necessary to palpate the cervix and upper vagina by rectal examination, taking specimens of the vaginal secretions for microscopy and culture. Examination of the anal region and rectum is as for men, but following the vaginal examination the abdomen is palpated for muscle guarding or for the detection of any lower abdominal masses, after which a bimanual examination is carried out to detect any swellings and areas of tenderness of the uterus and its appendages, as well as any masses within the pelvis.

From the patient's point of view the initial examination should normally be of that system which has produced symptoms, so that the general examination may proceed and/or follow that of the genitalia, and be of an extent determined by the findings of the genital examination, but will usually include the skin surfaces, mouth, eyes, lymph glands, joints, central nervous system and cardiovascular system, the routine being that of the individual clinician. Five ml of blood is taken for serological tests for syphilis and further specimens for *Herpesvirus* or *Chlamydia* antibody detection where necessary.

To eliminate the possibility of sexually transmitted diseases in both men and women a minimum of three complete examinations should be carried out, and in the case of women at least one should be during the immediate post-menstrual period, and serological tests be carried out for 3 months from risk of infection to eliminate the possibility of infection by syphilis. As soon as a patient is diagnosed as suffering from any of the sexually transmitted diseases he, or she, should be interviewed about all sexual contacts (see chapter 3, Medico-social Management).

FURTHER READING

Diagnostic Procedures for Viral and Rickettsial Diseases (1964). 3rd edn, Edited by E. H. Lenette & N. J. Schmidt. New York: American Public Health Association.

Enelow, A. J. & Swisher, S. N. (1972). *Interviewing and Patient Care,* Oxford University Press.

Harper, I. A. (1966). TRIC agent: characteristics and detection by laboratory methods. *British Journal of Venereal Diseases,* 42, 71.

Henderson, R. A., Rutherford, S., Phelps, J. A. & Robertson, P. (1970). Rapid direct immunofluorescent test for the gonococcus as a 'bench' procedure in venereal diseases clinics. *British Journal of Venereal Diseases,* 46, 205.

Mackenzie, D. W. R. (1966). *Symposium on Candida Infections,* p. 26. Edited by H. I. Winner & R. Henley. Edinburgh: Livingstone.

Martin, J. E. & Lester, A. (1971). Transgrow, a medium for transport and growth of *Neisseria gonorrhoeae* and *Neisseria meningitidis. H.S.H.M.A. Health Report,* 86, 30.

Rayner, C. F. K. (1968). Comparison of culture media for the growth of *Trichomonas vaginalis. British Journal of Venereal Diseases,* 44, 63.

Stuart, R. D., Tosback, S. R. & Patsula, R. M. (1954). Problem of transport of specimens for culture of gonococci. *Canadian Journal of Public Health,* 45, 73.

Wisdom, A. (1973). *A Colour Atlas of Venereology,* London: Wolfe Medical Books.

3. Public Health Cooperation and the Medico-Social Management of Sexually Transmitted Diseases

The medico-social management of the sexually transmitted diseases entails not only accuracy of diagnosis and permanency of cure, but, of equal or even greater importance from the Public Health point of view, the tracing and examination of each source of infection and all subsequent contacts. All those infected must be treated as rapidly and confidentially as was the propositus. This range of management, which is essential in the control of these contagious diseases, cannot be carried out by a private practitioner on his own. Even though a patient may pay in the expectation of getting better treatment and a greater certainty of confidentiality, it is most irresponsible and unethical to ignore those contacts at risk, whose disease will get worse with time and who, if promiscuous, will infect others. The responsibilities of those who are paid by individual patients are just as great as are those of doctors employed by public organizations.

PUBLIC HEALTH COOPERATION

The management of the medical and social aspects of sexually transmitted diseases cannot be the sole responsibility of the venereologist. To be effective it requires close collaboration between the public health administrators at governmental and local levels on the one hand and the venereologist and his colleagues on the other. In this way the greatest benefit accrues to the largest number of patients.

Governmental responsibilities

These are shared between the political and executive branches, the former devising policies based on information received from the executive branch, for the treatment and control of the diseases, the latter carrying out the policies, having put the case and the priority for the requirements to the political branch.

Financial. The government has to provide a service that is adequate for all its communities, and one that no citizen need forego because of the cost: with enough and conveniently sited clinics, properly equipped and adequately staffed with specialists and supporting staff, nursing, social and clerical, including sufficient training posts to provide a continuum of trained personnel, and last but not least having the support of adequate laboratory services.

Legislative. Laws have to be available to authorize an official service, which may include the certification of specialists, to protect the public against quackery, and other laws to combat prostitution, especially that which is organized. In Britain the confidentiality of the free service is accepted as basic to its success, but in certain circumstances some diseases need to be notified to the public health authorities and treatment made available to children and the handicapped, despite the fecklessness of their parents or guardians. In Britain, information can be passed to contact tracers without loss of medical confidence, while persons aged under 16 years can give consent for their own examination and treatment without parental permission, whenever it is considered they have sufficient mental capacity to know what that consent implies. In addition, those authorized to carry out contact tracing are protected against prosecution for slander or libel.

International cooperation. Governments have the responsibility for making, signing and ratifying international agreements on the availability of treatment for foreigners, such as the Brussels Agreement of 1924, the administration of which was taken over by the World Health Organization (WHO). In addition, the WHO and the International Labour Organization, which among other things concerns itself with the health of seamen, who export and import an appreciable amount of sexually transmitted diseases, need the financial support of every government to continue their eminently worth-while international services. International contact tracing is also the responsibility of governments, and they must ensure that the information is passed with alacrity and confidence, and is acted upon in a like manner.

Health education. It is a responsibility of each government to give its citizens every opportunity of leading a healthy life, and so to educate them. An uneducated public cannot be expected to cooperate with those attempting to help it. To inform the public effectively, all educational material must be presented in a manner that is understandable and acceptable. To do this efficiently a health education unit or division has to be set up within the executive, staffed by specialists in the fields of advertising, education and medicine. The health education material produced by such a department must be prepared in sufficient quantities to meet the requirements of all the local authorities. To inform those at risk of having sexually transmitted diseases, information of the location of the clinics and the times they are open should be widely available; publicity should be such that no-one is afraid of making use of the service, or of getting their consorts to attend for examination. In many areas, by telephoning a number listed in the directory under Hospital Services, Sexually Transmitted Diseases and Venereal Diseases, information can be obtained about local facilities, including the telephone numbers, addresses and times of the local clinics. Cautionary notices, warning of the dangers of indiscriminate promiscuity, should be widely displayed in those places where it is known that casual assignations are made. In the long term the most effective measure will be the education of school children from an early age, so that future generations will be unembarrassed and thoroughly informed in the responsibilities of sexuality, not merely of the techniques and physiology of sex and reproduction.

Epidemiological. The government needs to know the incidence and trends of the sexually transmitted diseases in each area, so that it can allocate, or reallocate, sufficient funds to maintain a proper service for each community all the time. In addition it has the responsibility of publishing the statistics, and the commentaries upon them, within a reasonable time. In this way, everyone, including the individual clinicians, may know the state of affairs in the country as a whole. Without published statistics it is impossible to evaluate the effects of current measures of disease control, so that changes from ineffective ones are delayed and those more effective are not taken up more vigorously.

Local authority responsibilities

The local health administrators are part of the executive of the local health authorities, which have powers delegated to them from the central government and obligations under the various Public Health Laws. Administrators have to get the support of the elected members of the various committees for the manner in which the various powers are to be used and the obligations implemented. Until 1974 in Britain the local authorities have been responsible for contact tracing, including interrogation, and supplied the personnel for this, as well as all the publicity for the clinical service, although the latter was under the Regional Hospital Boards. Because of this dichotomy the good-hearted cooperation and mutual understanding of the venereologist and the public health administrators has been required to make the service work efficiently. It is to be hoped that with the advent of an Integrated Health Service, collaboration will become even closer. With the general shortage of qualified staff, and the fact that the attributes of good interrogators and contact tracers are not always gauged by academic prowess, a number of appointments have to be made of so-called 'unqualified' social workers. It is the responsibility of the administrators, at their various levels, to place these workers into salary scales which are commensurate with their effectiveness. In this matter a lead from central governments is essential. Local authorities have the power to set up health education units which can make full use of the material prepared by the central government units, apart from producing their own material. Health education can be implemented in several ways: posters on public display, exhibitions and public lectures, apart from advertisements in the press, on the radio and television. The passive forms of education, or propaganda, when the public cannot avoid encounter with the material, are more effective than those which require active participation, such as exhibitions and lectures. In the latter the danger is of only 'preaching to the converted', while the real aim is to influence and inform those hitherto unconcerned or disinterested.

The clinician's responsibilities

Apart from personally maintaining a high standard of clinical practice, a venereologist must organize the clinical service, accepting his administrative responsibilities, so that the work is done smoothly. Some clinicians feel that administration is beneath their dignity, although of course, it is not; others lack a natural aptitude for it, but if it does not make perfect, practice does improve ability. The venereologist is responsible for providing evidence of the need for extra facilities and also that those in use are being used effectively. Lacking this evidence administrators at all levels will be unable to ensure favourable political decisions regarding finance, as they often have to overcome reluctance, or even antagonism, by those who express antipathy towards sufferers of sexually transmitted diseases. The administrators must put a very strong case, and be well briefed. Statistics must be collected as accurately as possible: alone they are an indication of work done, in comparison with others and over a period of time, they indicate trends of the various diseases, and the scope of various facilities needed.

Each venereologist is pivotal to recruitment into the specialty; without his example as a clinician, enthusiasm as a teacher and pride in his vocation, no amount of government finance will fill the junior posts in his department.

The venereologist has several responsibilities in health education. He should be available to give advice to those producing educational material on the facts or points which should be publicized, and indicate any special 'target sites', where special material may prove effective. He should teach those who are going to be instructors in health education, explaining and discussing with them the background of the sexually transmitted diseases, their cure and the risk of promiscuity and the personal responsibility needed to cope with sexuality, so that they can pass on the information, in a confident and unembarrassed manner. Probably the greatest responsibility of the venereologist in the field of health education is his instruction of medical students, undergraduates and postgraduates, not so much to make them specialists as to train them to recognize the sexually transmitted diseases as such, and to appreciate their significance within the sphere of sexuality. Hitherto, all too few doctors have been able to discuss sexuality with their patients, and its associated problems, in an unembarrassed and unemotional manner. The need for education of the medical profession is greater than that for the public in general. As yet very few universities or medical schools, if any, have been persuaded of the deficiencies in their courses of instruction. Venereologists have the unpleasant, but important duty of reiterating the deficiencies of instruction in sexuality, and the effects of its misuse, illegitimacy and sexually transmitted diseases, to the deans and medical faculties, many of whom do not appreciate the problems.

MEDICO-SOCIAL MANAGEMENT

Medico-social management entails more than the diagnosis and treatment of patients. It includes the tracing of contacts, case holding and efforts to get defaulters to reattend. This type of management requires a specialized team including venereologists, nurses, technicians, social workers and health visitors, an integration of hospital service and public health staffs. In practice the work can only be carried out by departments set up specifically for this purpose.

Contact tracing

The aim of contact tracing is to get all contacts examined and treated as quickly as possible and so prevent further spread of infection, especially to 'innocent' people.

The needs for effective contact tracing. This relies on the accuracy of diagnosis, which is of paramount importance. Before patients will tell the truth about their contacts they have to have faith in the clinic, and this they can only gain from the way they have been treated themselves. This goodwill takes time to build up, but with any mismanagement is soon dissipated.

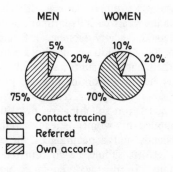

Fig. 4 The sources of patients with gonorrhoea.

Apart from accuracy of diagnosis, effective contact tracing is based on the results of an interview. Sufficient information has to be obtained to identify every contact, if possible. Unfortunately this does not always happen. Names and addresses are usually available of husbands, wives and sweethearts, and occasionally of friends or acquaintances; sometimes their telephone numbers are known. When, as often happens, these facts are unknown the forename or nickname and a description of the contact may be of great value; the height should be recorded as a measurement; the build can vary from fat, plump, well built, slim, thin to skinny, never accepting the word 'medium', although buxom may be of use when appropriate. The description of hair may be a problem because of the popularity of wigs, but the colour, length and style should be noted; age should be recorded, although it is usually underestimated. Information about casual contacts should include the meeting place, the job, occupation or whether unemployed; the type and style of the clothes worn; if a prostitute how much was charged. In addition, any special characteristics that might be of help in identification, although such things as tattoos, birthmarks, scars, speech and accent, drinking habits and friends are rarely noticed by patients. It is also useful to know where the patient was infected and, if a foreigner, his nationality and colour, because some women only consort with men of a certain ethnic group. All this information is best recorded on a proforma or special card at the time of interview.

A number of contacts are unknown, but the descriptions of some do fit known promiscuous people who have attended previously. Over the years each department builds up a dossier of promiscuous people, usually women. Information for this is compiled from the descriptions of those who have attended, together with their habits, haunts and family background; from reports of other health visitors of possible problem families in their districts; from newspaper reports of women drunk and disorderly, in court for soliciting or prostitution; also from information supplied by women already attending, who often discuss their friends and acquaintances. In each area all the contact tracing efforts should be coordinated and information collected centrally. In this way contacts named by patients attending different clinics can be sought more quickly and efforts are not duplicated.

Interview. Interviewing of both male and female patients is usually more effectively carried out by a woman. The majority of patients interrogated are men, who, having had a genital examination, blood taken for serological testing and probably an intramuscular injection, all under conditions of personal stress, do tend to relax when removed from the clinical atmosphere into the presence of a friendly and presentable woman, whose age appears irrelevant. Under these circumstances patients give information unobtainable by the doctor in the consulting-room and the nurse or technician in the treatment-room. The psychological reaction is probably the same as that used in espionage, first the pain then the kindness. A man with gonorrhoea should be told that the woman who infected him is probably asymptomatic and does not know that she is infectious. All patients should be reassured about the confidence of the information being requested, that the contacts will not know who gave the information, and that the tracing will be done without embarrassment or publicity. Married patients, who may have infected their spouses, but dare not admit to extramarital intercourse, should be reassured that the spouse can be examined and treated without necessarily being told the nature of the disease. It is not the duty of a venereologist or the members of his staff to proffer such information which may cause the break-up of a marriage, shaky though it may be. Urethritis may be described as a 'chill on the bladder' or a 'bladder infection', cervicitis as a 'woman's complaint'. If the spouse does ask a direct question, then it must be answered truthfully, but only rarely is such a question asked. There is no doubt that a number of infected wives have a pretty good idea of the significance of the infection but, as long as the truth is not thrust upon them, can avoid having to face the implications. They are usually in a very difficult position. If they leave their husbands who is going to maintain them, and what will happen to the children? The vast majority of marriages recover from an isolated episode, most husbands having learnt their lesson, but may not if repeated. Finally, contact tracing efforts must be made with all possible speed, to prevent further infections and to locate the contact before she moves to another address.

Methods of contact tracing. Whenever possible the innocent partner of a steady relationship, married or otherwise, should be examined by appointment at a special 'diagnostic' centre rather than in the normal clinics, the patient taking or sending the partner. Some patients bring their contacts to a clinic, others take 'follow-up cards' which they give to contacts who bring them to the clinics. These cards should have the addresses, 'phone numbers and times of the clinics on one side, and on the other such names of the contact as are known, the clinic number of the patient and his diagnosis in code. Visits are made by contact tracers, either social workers or nurses from the community nursing service, when a description fits someone already known, when a patient does not want to approach a certain contact himself or when a spouse has failed to keep an appointment. Visiting is useful in that information is obtained about the home circumstances otherwise unobtainable, such as friends found at the home, who may be patients already attending. On other occasions visits are arranged in peripheral areas by the local specialist in community medicine who may even arrange for the contact to see him in his office, on which occasion an appointment is made for her to attend a clinic. In some cases, when a contact is known to frequent a certain coffee bar, café or public house, she may be approached in these premises by a contact tracer. On very rare occasions general practitioners may be requested to help, but often this is resented by the contacts who do not wish to 'lose face' in the sight of their doctor, nor are many general practitioners happy to appear to be spying on behalf of a hospital department. Sometimes contacts are found to be in hospital, women with salpingitis, not infrequently diagnosed as appendicitis, men with epididymitis and both sexes with rashes of secondary syphilis under investigation, or condylomata being treated as haemorrhoids or condylomata acuminata in surgical wards.

Other methods of obtaining contacts include 'cluster testing' of close associates of patients, the screening of groups considered to be at special risk of having a sexually transmitted disease, girls in remand homes and approved schools and women in prison, or other groups not necessarily at special risk, immigrants, food handlers, blood donors, couples before marriage and women during pregnancy. All these methods do produce a number of cases that otherwise would not have been discovered for some time, but the frequency in some groups is minimal. In some countries certain sexually transmitted diseases are notifiable and it is claimed that this helps in contact tracing procedures.

Case holding

The success of the medico-social management of sexually transmitted diseases in any area depends on the faith the local promiscuous people, especially the highly promiscuous, have in the clinic staff. This faith takes a long time to build up and it can be lost quickly by the mismanagement of these patients. There must be no moralizing and they must be made to feel free to attend for a check-up at any time, when they should be able to expect an accurate and rapid, if not immediate, diagnosis. They should not be pestered by unnecessary default efforts, only being sought when it is believed that they have not been cured of a disease or have been reinfected, the effort being made by a visit or telephone call, the matter being treated as urgent.

At the first visit the doctor should explain the diagnosis, unless this is being withheld, the treatment and the need for surveillance, all in such plain language that each patient can understand. Whenever instructions are given, such as no alcohol to be taken for a period of time following the treatment of urethritis, all the members of the staff must take the same line. Everyone must adopt a sympathetic, but amoral, attitude towards the patient, neither condemning nor congratulating, mainly reassuring that cure is certain if treatment and instructions are carried out. As painful handling of patients is a cause of default, the techniques of all the members of the staff must be of the highest possible standard. An amount of default can be prevented by having a social worker available in the clinics who provides a ready ear to the patients who can tell of their various troubles. Many of those on prolonged surveillance, at intervals of three or more months, welcome a reminder note informing them that their next appointment is due; this can be arranged with individual patients.

Default. Default, the antithesis of case holding, is often caused by misunderstandings between the patient and the staff, occasionally by mishandling, possibly by an inferred criticism or by painful examination or treatment. Default is more common in clinics inconveniently sited, away from public transport, with entrances overlooked by the general public, in the basements of hospitals or tucked away in the corner of hospital grounds, and when the sessions are held at unsuitable hours. Attendance by appointment may cut down the rate of default and is more convenient for the staff, but some new patients may not feel able to wait a day or so for an appointment and will go to an 'open' clinic where they know they will be seen, if not immediately, at least during the current session. Badly organized appointment systems, when clinics are overbooked, do cause default among those not prepared to wait long beyond the time of their appointment. Patients in peripatetic occupations, such as merchant seamen and long distance lorry drivers, cannot always attend regularly, and those who have defaulted in the past usually do so again.

Default efforts. Attempts to get patients to return from default should be taken rapidly; the longer the delay in making an effort the worse the response. Male patients with gonorrhoea should only require a single default letter, unless syphilis is suspected or further information is needed about contacts. Patients on surveillance following treatment for syphilis should have further letters. Visits should be made whenever untreated syphilis is suspected, treatment uncompleted and, if possible, for all women. Default letters are not very successful, they are impersonal and a proportion of patients have given false names and addresses. Visits are much more effective: a personal interest is being shown, although individual patients may not appreciate this interest, and at the same time the visitor can learn much about the defaulter. Those doing default visiting must know the reason for the visit, and be able to explain this to the patient. When a defaulter does return he/she must be made to feel that they are welcomed back, and although the doctor may point out the dangers of default none of the other members of the staff proffers any criticism. Indeed the nursing, technical and social staffs must always appear to be the patients' friends without appearing to criticize the doctors.

THE POSITION IN GREAT BRITAIN

The reasons for the success in disease control in Great Britain can be summarized as follows: free treatment for all is provided in special out-patient departments situated throughout the country. Attendance is voluntary, there is no enforced treatment; treatment is confidential, there is no nominal notification; all patients are under the care of a specialist in sexually transmitted diseases; all sexually transmitted diseases, including those labelled venereal, are treated.

Under the National Health Service Act of 1947, Venereology was recognized as a specialty in its own right, all specialties having the same career and salary structure, all consultants having equal status. Because of this, venereologists, or more recently specialists in sexually transmitted diseases, have become accepted as the local experts in the management of sexually transmitted diseases.

The public has found out, over the years, that the best treatment is obtained in the special clinics where full case histories and careful clinical examinations enable complications to be diagnosed and treated as such.

The medico-social management of the sexually transmitted diseases is provided by a specialized team; on the medical side, one of specialist doctors, nurses and technicians, including trainees, and an adequate laboratory service; on the social side, one of community nurses, social and welfare workers. All the team try to treat patients with care and consideration. If patients are dealt with in this way during diagnosis and treatment, they are more likely to be forthcoming with information during interviews concerning their sexual contacts.

Contact tracing efforts are based on accuracy of diagnosis and no treatment without diagnosis. Interviewing of patients is carried out in private and all information obtained is treated as confidential. Later 'white lies' may be told to 'innocent' partners who are usually examined and, if necessary, treated in premises apart from the recognised clinic.

The effectiveness of these measures in Great Britain is reflected in the low incidence of syphilis and gonorrhoea, compared with elsewhere. In fact, the control of the other sexually transmitted diseases now poses a greater problem to the Health Service in Great Britain than does that of the venereal diseases themselves.

FURTHER READING

Bernfield, W. K. (1967). Medical professional secrecy with special reference to venereal diseases. *British Journal of Venereal Diseases*, 43, 53.

Brown, W. J., Donohue, J. F., Axnick, N. W., Blount, J. H., Ewen, N. H. & Jones, O. G. (1970). *Syphilis and Other Venereal Diseases*. London: Oxford University Press.

Dalzell-Ward, A. J. (1969). Britain's venereal disease education for high-risk, age and cultural groups. *Medical Officer*, 121, 3.

Hammar, H. & Ljungberg, L. (1972). Factors affecting contact tracing of gonorrhoea. *Acta dermato-venereologica*, Stockholm, 52, 233.

Johnson, D. W., Holmes, K. K., Kvale, P. A., Halverson, C. W. & Hirsch, W. P. (1969). Evaluation of gonorrhoea case finding in the chronically-infected female. *American Journal of Epidemiology*, 90, 438.

Ministry of Health. 'Health Education' Report by a Joint Committee of the Scottish and Central Health Service Councils (1964). H.M.S.O., London, S.O. Code No. 32–523.

Moerloose, J. de & Rahm, H. (1964). A survey of venereal disease legislation in Europe. *Acta dermato-venereologica*, *Stockholm*, 44, 146.

Webster, B. (1966). Teaching of venereal diseases in medical schools throughout the world. Preliminary report. *British Journal of Venereal Diseases*, 42, 132.

Wells, B. W. P. & Schofield, C. B. S. (1970). 'Target' sites for anti-V.D. propaganda. *Health Bulletin. Department of Health for Scotland*, XXVIII, 1, 75.

4. The Sociological and Psychological Background to the Sexually Transmitted Diseases

Following the social upheaval due to the industrial revolution, societies in the developed countries remained fairly static until the 1914-18 War. During this period there was little movement within the social classes and, except for migration, the majority of people lived and died in the districts where they were born. During the past fifty years, however, there has been an increasing mobility of people in search of better opportunities as commerce has changed, the old industries declining and new ones developing, and this has caused a breakdown in the established class structure. These processes have become accelerated and world-wide over the past twenty-five years as the developing countries have become progressively urbanized, their rural communities declining. As a consequence the young no longer accept

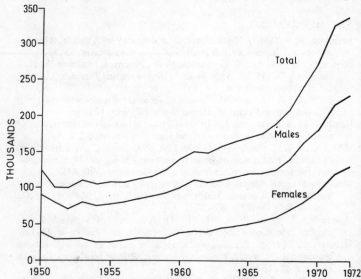

Fig. 5 New patients attending special clinics in Britain, 1950-1972; totals, males and females.

uncritically the standards of religious or political ideals, and sexual morals set for them by their elders. This is especially so when the young have moved away from the elders of their own tribe, clan or community.

The questioning of standards has resulted in less hypocrisy but a loss of security, since new solutions must be sought by individuals, each one tested personally, and when found unsound later rejected, until eventually a satisfactory answer is discovered. In many cases the old rejected standards have yet to be replaced by the new, and the 'new morality' remains in a state of flux. Many of the facets of current societies predispose towards an increase in promiscuity, which affects social classes, religious and political persuasions indiscriminately. Promiscuity takes several forms: it may be indiscriminate, when risks are taken with unknown and casual partners, or with discrimination when only with friends; it may be persistent, when risks are taken regularly, or intermittent, when they are taken at intervals, often only very occasionally. The risks may be concurrent, with several partners during one period of time or sequential, with one partner only during any given period. The increase in the incidence of sexually transmitted diseases is a result of the increase in indiscriminate promiscuity which is the basic problem, the acquisition of a disease being merely fortuitous.

THE SOCIOLOGICAL BACKGROUND

Many of the current aspects of society in the developed and developing countries predispose to indiscriminate promiscuity, and so to a consequent increase in sexually transmitted disease. Within a closed community promiscuity is not associated with disease, unless it is introduced from outside. Promiscuity appears to be encouraged by certain aspects of current societies, mobility, addiction, materialism, permissiveness, mass information and effective contraception.

Mobility. Apart from emigration and immigration, especially of single people rather than of family groups, in most countries there is a persistent migration from rural communities and the smaller towns into the larger ones where, because of insufficient accommodation to cope with the influx, overcrowding and slum development, including the sharing of rooms, has become a serious problem. Many of the single people are lonely and, because sexual standards deteriorate when away from the supervision of the home communities, a number of them have indiscriminate and casual sexual intercourse.

Addiction. In Britain addiction, or rather the persistent over-consumption of drugs, is mainly associated with alcohol. In Scotland the amount of drunkenness and alcoholism is a matter of grave concern. Elsewhere, and under different circumstances other drugs may be the major problem; it is largely a matter of availability. The relationship between alcohol and promiscuity in Britain is well established, over 90 per cent of casual contacts being met within or outside bars or public houses, these being the only places where strangers meet and make temporary friends, while the inhibitions are clouded by alcohol. Sixty-four per cent of male patients reported that alcohol made women more willing to have sex with them while 54 per cent of female patients stated that alcohol made them more relaxed and, in 48 per cent, increased their interest in and enjoyment of sex. The association between other drugs and promiscuity is less close, but in one clinic both male and female drug takers had had, on average, 37 per cent more sex partners than non-drug takers of the same age. In Glasgow, of the 295 new patients aged from 16 to 24 years inclusive who were interviewed between 1970 and 1972, 44 (15 per cent) admitted to having taken non-therapeutic drugs within a week of attending. In all, 43 per cent of 136 males and 36 per cent of 159 females had taken drugs at some time and usually more than one drug. Of the male drug takers, 93 per cent had used cannabis, 43 per cent lysergic acid diethylamide (LSD), 34 per cent amphetamines and oral barbiturates, 19 per cent tranquillisers and 12 per cent intravenous heroin. Of the females, 79 per cent had taken cannabis, 34 per cent LSD, 29 per cent oral barbiturates, 22 per cent amphetamines, 14 per cent tranquillisers and 12 per cent intravenous heroin. None had used intravenous barbiturates. It is of interest that in 1970, prior to the local voluntary control in the prescription of amphetamines and barbiturates, the incidence of misuse of both these drugs was 40 per cent for males and 50 per cent and 65 per cent respectively for females. Cannabis in men and women, and the barbiturates (Mandrax especially) in women were usually, but LSD only occasionally, associated with an improvement in the quality of sexual intercourse. In men, this was reported in the following order, increase in sexual drive, a prolongation of coitus and a heightened climax, and in women firstly relaxation, with a greater chance of achieving orgasm, which was heightened, coitus being prolonged.

Materialism. Many societies are considered materialistic. An undue emphasis is laid on getting things now and paying later or attempting to get something for nothing. These aspects are reflected in the amount of hire purchase and the increase in gambling. In addition, nutrition has improved, ill-health decreased and sexual maturity occurs at an earlier age than before. With current wage structures the young have attained financial independence, and their parents thus lost this form of control. Some parents, who remember from their childhood the depressions of the 1920s and 1930s when they lacked material things, have overcompensated with their children and provided a suberabundance of those things which they had lacked. To do this, often both parents have had to work all day, and this, together with the fact that many go out again in the evenings, has caused a deprivation in the home, spiritual rather than material, but of much greater danger to the young.

Permissiveness. Many societies are now permissive in regard to sexual matters. In most of them there is less stigma to marriage breakdown, illegitimacy, pre- and extra-marital intercourse and homosexuality. These may well be considered enlightened and humane attitudes, but in the presence of an increasing amount of propaganda denigrating sexual continence before and outside marriage, including the examples set by certain 'peer groups', can cause the less sophisticated to act in a manner which will lead to unhappiness. The groups who reap the benefit are those 'personalities' made prominent by the mass media who, in an atmosphere of declining censorship, extol permissiveness and counter opposition by labelling their antagonists as 'reactionaries', a vogue word having tremendous defamatory capabilities. The effects of all this propaganda, much of it with solid commercial backing, is to encourage a generalized increase in indiscriminate promiscuity.

'Mass information'. Because of the mass media, people in all walks of life the whole world over can now see how those with more money and opportunity manage their lives. Not unnaturally this brings about an amount of discontent, and it has now become apparent to all that 'those at the top' do not always live the exemplary lives they were supposed to lead, and which they have encouraged upon the masses. In addition, a small number of

people, not necessarily representative of the majority of opinion, are able to exert an undue influence through their positions, either in control of, or by their exposure through, the mass media. In the atmosphere of permissiveness some of them do proffer promiscuous behaviour as being 'biologically normal' and therefore acceptable. Their message is accepted uncritically by all too many of those lacking the discrimination of the more worldly wise. The antibiotic era, which is now over 25 years old, and the wide publicity of the effectiveness of such drugs, has engendered an unwarranted confidence as to their universal effectiveness. There is now little fear, if any, in the sexually transmitted diseases and a consequent carelessness in promiscuous sexual behaviour.

Contraception. The advent of effective contraceptive measures, the gestogen pills and intra-uterine devices, which lack the barrier provided by the condom, have given women freedom from unwanted pregnancies but not from the sexually transmitted diseases. Seventy-eight per cent of female, but only 16 per cent of male, patients cited 'the Pill' as one of the reasons for the reported current increase in sexual activity. As these measures are under the control of women themselves the whole relationship between the sexes has been altered, and many men bitterly resent it, women now having an equal opportunity to become promiscuous. It is doubtful if women will exercise this freedom as indiscriminately as have men in the past, but already changes in the pattern of promiscuity have become apparent, more women becoming intermittently promiscuous than before. It may well mean that prostitution will disappear when a sufficient proportion of men are able to have sexual intercourse with the increasing number of women who are somewhat promiscuous. This will slow down the rate of transmission of the sexually transmitted diseases and may facilitate control measures, but the greater the number of men undergoing vasectomy, the latest generally accepted contraceptive measure, the more the situation will revert to its former position.

Social patterns. The various social factors mentioned, among others, cause differences in the distribution of gonorrhoea as far as age, sex, social and marital status and source of infection are concerned, from one area to another and from one time to another in any one area. To illustrate this, it might be helpful to compare the results of a study carried out on patients treated for gonorrhoea in Glasgow during 1972 with that of 1967. In both studies, note was made from the clinic records of the age, sex, social class, or that of the husband in the case of married women, and of the source of infection in relation to marital status. There were 600 men and 400 women in the 1972 study, 495 men and 280 women in 1967. Differences in age distribution between the men and women attending in 1972 are shown in Table 1, the controls being the population of Glasgow.

Table 1 The percentage distribution by age groups of men and women suffering from gonorrhoea in 1972

	Number of patients	Age group (years)					
		15–19	20–29	30–39	40–49	50–59	60–69
Men Patients	600	12.0	56·8	19·3	7·7	3·2	1·0
Men Controls		13·1	21·2	14·7	17·2	18·2	15·6
Women Patients	400	30·75	51·0	12·25	4·25	1·25	0·5
Women Controls		11·8	20·0	14·5	17·1	19·2	17·4

In the five years between the studies the average age fell by 1·48 years for the men and by 2·34 years for the women, but in both the main differences in the distribution between the sexes were found among the teenagers and those in their forties. (From henceforth, 1967 figures will be quoted in parenthesis). Teenage girls had two and a half times (80 per cent more) and boys only 90 per cent (two-thirds) of the anticipated proportion of gonorrhoea. Men in their forties had 45 per cent (two-thirds) and women 25 per cent (one-third) of the expected proportion. In their twenties, the years of greatest sexual activity, both sexes had relatively similar incidences, in both studies, of over two and a half times the expected proportion. In their thirties, men accounted for 30 per cent in excess (20 per cent more) and women 20 per cent less (20 per cent more) of the anticipated proportion. Only 4·2 per cent (4·1 per cent) of gonorrhoea was found in the 33·8 per cent (30·7 per cent) of men aged 50 years and over and 1·75 per cent (3·0 per cent) in the 36·6 per cent (34·8 per cent) of women.

While promiscuity continues to affect all the social strata in Glasgow, the reported prevalence of gonorrhoea does vary between the social classes as defined by the Registrar General, and in women there remains a further variation depending on marital status, as is shown in Table 2, the controls consisting of the male working population of Glasgow.

Table 2 The percentage distribution by social class of men and of women, married or otherwise, with gonorrhoea

	Number of patients	Social class				
		Class I	Class II	Class III	Class IV	Class V
Men	600	3·3	12·5	42·5	20·0	21·7
Married women	115	3·5	7·8	40·9	17·4	30·4
Unmarried women	285	0·4	8·4	40·0	11·6	39·6
Total males in Glasgow	–	3·2	9·0	54·1	20·4	13·3

In social class I, the proportion of all men and of married women approximated that of the working community (as before), and there was one unmarried woman. (None in 1967.) There was an excess of men, mainly unmarried, in class II and almost as many women, married or otherwise (fewer married in 1967) as expected, while in class III there were fewer men and women than expected (as in 1967). In class IV there were as many men, (fewer in 1967) but fewer women (as in 1967) than expected. These findings in classes III and IV probably reflect the dwindling remnants of 'middle class morality'. There was an excess of men, and a marked excess of women in class V especially of the unmarried (as in 1967), an increasing proportion of whom appeared to have no means of gainful employment.

Sources of infection. The proportions of the various types of marital status differ in the two studies. In 1972 the decrease in married patients is matched by increases in men formerly married and in single women. Of the men, only 28 per cent were married (38 per cent in 1967) while 13 per cent were formerly married (5 per cent) and 59 per cent were single (57 per cent). As far as the women are concerned only 29 per cent were married (39 per cent), 14 per cent were formerly married (14 per cent) while 57 per cent were single (47 per cent).

Table 3 The percentage source of infection by sex and marital status

Marital status	Number of patients	Source of infection			
		Marital	Friend	Casual	Prostitute
Men					
Married	168	8	22	60	10
Formerly married*	80	–	15	75	10
Single	352	–	21	77	2
Women					
Married	115	80	15	5	–
Formerly married*	57	–	67	33	–
Single	228	–	35	65	–

*Formerly married includes those separated, divorced or widowed.

Only 5·3 per cent of men were infected by prostitutes (14·2 per cent) and single men only rarely, but 72 per cent were infected by casual amateurs (70 per cent), the proportions varying from 60 per cent of married men (55 per cent) to 77 per cent of the single (80 per cent). Over one fifth of the men were infected by friends (less than an eighth), the married 22 per cent (16 per cent), the single 21 per cent (10 per cent) and the formerly married 15 per cent (10 per cent), while 8 per cent of married men were infected by their wives (9 per cent). In all, over 77 per cent of infections in men were due to indiscriminate promiscuity (85 per cent).

The vast proportion of married women, 80 per cent, were infected by their husbands (85 per cent), 67 per cent of those formerly married were infected by friends (63 per cent) and 65 per cent of the single by casual consorts (70 per cent). As before, about twice as many of those married, past or present, were infected by friends rather than casual consorts, the reverse holding good for single women. Forty-three per cent of infections in women were due to indiscriminate promiscuity (40 per cent).

A marked decrease in the incidence of venereal disease has been reported from communist China where, as an integral part of their political philosophy, sexual continence and marriage deferred until the late 20's has been vigorously encouraged, if not made mandatory. Possibly of greater importance was the social rehabilitation, during the cultural revolution, of the prostitutes, hitherto the main source of venereal disease in that country.

These methods of disease control appear to have been effective during a period of revolutionary fervour and when foreigners were initially excluded from China. With the influx of visitors from abroad, which must follow the increase in trade and cultural exchange with other countries, there is a grave risk that China will experience an increase in the incidence of venereal and of sexually transmitted diseases. It would appear unwise of the Chinese public health authorities to disband their facilities for the treatment of sexually transmitted diseases, especially in those areas where foreigners will be visiting. In addition, they must prepare for the time when the current revolutionary spirit has waned during the period of consolidation by generations that never know or experienced the actual revolution. This is the stage or period in a country's evolution when boredom is liable to creep in and with it sexual promiscuity among other manifestations of antisocial behaviour. This series of events has already been seen in the USSR where the sons and daughters of the revolutionaries have not behaved with the dedication and moral behaviour of their parents. Boredom and the lack of some positive aim in life, ethnic, political, social or religious predisposes towards sexual promiscuity in any society.

THE PSYCHOLOGICAL BACKGROUND

A century or less ago 'ladies' merely 'submitted' to coitus. This was the period of the great 'dual morality' hypocrisy when promiscuity on the part of a man was only frowned upon but in a woman was considered an outrage to society. Today the 'dual morality' is no longer accepted. Along with the development of the permissive society have come changed attitudes to sexuality, and it is now acknowledged as normal that sex should be enjoyable to both men and women, especially when effective contraceptive techniques are readily available.

From the psychological point of view it is not surprising that sexual freedom has led to an increase in promiscuity, the vast majority being intermittent and with discrimination, and not associated with sexually transmitted disease. Not all of these casual sexual relationships, however, are satisfactory. While fear probably only plays a small part, a number of ordinary and unsophisticated people still have strong inhibitions, which some call conscience, sufficient to prevent the achievement of an orgasm. These people may have to await the development of a stable relationship before sex becomes enjoyable, while the less inhibited can enjoy each episode. Promiscuity in the single, or unattached, is often due to loneliness, when a relationship of instant intimacy is taken up with a casual acquaintance, and almost always followed by immediate parting. Promiscuity by one of a couple is often due to an imbalance in sexuality, the one more highly sexed becoming promiscuous, unless both partners have insight into the problem and can make adjustments.

Persistent and indiscriminate promiscuity is quite a different matter, and when extreme may be considered psycho-pathological. In men it is usually associated with immaturity and poor emotional adjustment. Although often extroverted, these men find great difficulty in forming strong interpersonal relation-ships. They tend to be dull and lack self-confidence, often they appear to have failed to achieve their own ambitions, but are not able to rationalize their failings and may use their higher sexuality in an attempt to prove themselves superior. Rarely does this succeed, and their reputed prowess is not always confirmed. A number of these men start as social drinkers, but often become heavy drinkers, possibly as prowess declines, and later may become alcoholics. In other circumstances they will just as easily take to drugs when they are available.

Persistently promiscuous women are also immature and often are looking for 'love', seeking emotional support and comfort rather than physical satisfaction. Usually they are feckless, never preparing for the future, and, because of their lack of responsi-bility, do not hold jobs. They tend to be emotionally facile and often tell lies needlessly, sometimes living in a dream world of their own. Under these circumstances it is not surprising that many of them drink to excess, take to drugs or both, and that a high proportion of them are psychotic.

The differences in the incidence of the sexually transmitted diseases between male and female teenagers has already been mentioned, boys having a lower, and girls a much higher incidence than expected. This might be explained by the ways in which they 'revolt'. Boys usually join gangs and start drinking, or possibly taking drugs, and within the security of the herd, and under the influence of drink, carry out petty larcenies, vandalism and violence against the person, often in such a foolhardy manner as to bring them in contact with the law. Sex plays only a minor role in the majority of cases, but if the boy is a 'drop out', or made to feel one, then sex may play a more dominant role. Girls in revolt run away from home; then they become promiscuous, sometimes attached to a gang of boys or group of single men, possible immigrants, and then take to drink or drugs. Pregnancy not infrequently follows, and this may well be wanted. Many of these girls want to have a baby, but more as a doll than as a child who will have to be cared for and looked after. As a consequence of their promiscuity they have a high rate of sexually transmitted disease and, as a result of this or a pregnancy, may be rejected by the gang or men. At, or before this time, and especially if they are on drugs, suicide attempts may be made. Some are gestures in search of attention, others are deadly serious and whenever discovered should never be taken lightly. These five entities, leaving home, promiscuity, pregnancy, sexually transmitted disease and suicide attempts form a pattern of behaviour or syndrome and, whenever it is found incomplete, the missing entities should be anticipated.

Personality patterns

It is recognized that an individual's reactions in any situation are governed in part by his or her personality. Among the instruments available to define the various types of personality are questionnaires such as Eysenck's Personality Inventory (EPI), which measures the two major dimensions or personality, extroversion and neuroticism, and Eysenck's PEN Inventory which, in addition, measures psychoticism. These questionnaires are completed by the subjects themselves, and from the results obtained an association or difference between various groups of patients can be found, which can be assessed statistically.

The aim of psychological investigations, carried out on patients with sexually transmitted diseases, is to find out why they behave as they do and, by learning more about their motivations, to be better able to help them, and to advise on effective methods of disease control. Using the EPI and PEN questionnaires different patterns of personality have become apparent between the sexes, within sexes according to the source of infections, whether or not the patients completed surveillance and, in males, whether they were hetero- or homosexual.

Male patients differ from the normal population only in that they are significantly more extroverted, but female patients are more introverted and significantly more neurotic, in addition to which they score highly for psychoticism. With regard to the source of infection, innocent husbands tend to be introverted but do not score highly on neuroticism or psychoticism as do the innocent wives to a marked degree. These women differ from the normal population in neuroticism and psychoticism as much as do the promiscuous women infected by casual consorts, the latter scoring more highly on extroversion. Most of the men infected by casual consorts are not highly promiscuous; they do not score highly on neuroticism or psychoticism but they are extroverted. In both sexes the group nearest to the normal population, from which they do not differ significantly, are those infected by friends. An amount of neuroticism found among these women can be accounted for by the fact that the term, 'friend', may be applied to any relationship from being engaged to having met twice, and some of the women might well have been included in the casual group. In general men tend to play down the relationship while women upgrade it.

Among men, those defaulting have significantly higher scores for neuroticism and psychoticism than those completing surveillance, who are apparently normal. Quite a different pattern appears in women, default being associated with extroversion but not with neuroticism or psychoticism. Male patients who are drug takers, but not females, have significantly higher scores for neuroticism and also anxiety as measured by the IPAT anxiety scale than non-drug taking patients.

Homosexual male patients only differed from heterosexual males in that they scored highly for neuroticism, more especially those classified as 'passive'. Homosexuals were divided arbitrarily into 'active' or 'passive' groups according to the type of risk which had caused their attendance, although the majority stated that they took part in other forms of sexual behaviour. The 'active' homosexuals were somewhat less extroverted than the 'passives', who had higher scores for neuroticism.

What do these findings tell us and what use can we make of them? First they explain the behaviour of some patients; that a number of 'erring' husbands are extroverted and commit adultery, following domestic crises, when their wives are introverted and neurotic, this dissimilarity being the prime cause of the marriage breakdown, the reverse holding good in the case of the 'erring' wife. Secondly it confirms that homosexual patients tend towards neuroticism, that only an amount of extroversion is needed in a man to enable him to pick-up an unknown woman and persuade her to have coitus on their first, and possibly only, meeting, but that it needs a significant amount of neuroticism and psychoticism, together with some extroversion on her behalf, for her to accept his advances. It is not surprising that these women, who have sex with casual consorts, are considered abnormal, because they have had to reject the conventions of society. The high degree of neuroticism and psychoticism found in female patients and in male defaulters indicate that these groups require explanations in excess of those given to other patients to impress upon them the necessity to complete treatment and surveillance. It must be accepted that they do not necessarily think as do the normal or the non-promiscuous population, and allowances must be made for this in all instructions and propaganda issued. They cannot be expected to react favourably to advice that would be accepted by more normal groups.

Use can be made of these findings in the field of health education, apart from within the clinic itself, especially in the sex education given to schoolchildren before they take an active interest in sex. Those girls having a high rating for neuroticism and psychoticism, and the boys who are extroverted, require extra and specialized sex instruction in the responsibilities of sexuality and the dangers of its misuse, in an attempt to prevent them from becoming indiscriminately promiscuous.

FURTHER READING

Brecher, R. & Brecher, E., editors (1968). *An Analysis of Human Sexual Response.* London: Panther Books.

Catterall, R. D. (1965). Venereal disease and teenagers. *Practitioner,* 195, 620.

Geiger, J. (1973). Behind the bamboo curtain. World Medicine, 9, No. 22, 15.

Idsøe, O. & Guthe, T. (1967). The rise and fall of the treponematoses—I. Ecological aspects of international trends in venereal syphilis. *British Journal of Venereal Diseases,* 43, 227.

Idsøe, O., Kiraly, K. & Causse, G. (1973). Venereal disease and treponematoses—the epidemiological situation and the WHO's control programme. *World Health Organization Chronicle,* 27, 410.

Juhlin, L. (1968). Factors influencing the spread of gonorrhoea—I. Educational and social behaviour. *Acta dermato-venereologia, Stockholm,* **48,** 75.

Juhlin, L. (1968). Factors influencing the spread of gonorrhoea—II. Sexual behaviour at different ages. *Acta dermato-venereologia, Stockholm,* **48,** 82.

Juhlin, L. & Liden, S. (1969). Influence of contraceptive gestogen pills on sexual behaviour and the spread of gonorrhoea. *British Journal of Venereal Diseases,* **45,** 321.

Linken, A. (1968). A study of drug taking among young people attending a clinic for venereal diseases. *British Journal of Venereal Diseases,* **44,** 337.

Linken, A. & Wiener, R. B. D. (1970). Promiscuity and contraception in a group of patients attending a clinic for venereal diseases. *British Journal of Venereal Diseases,* **46,** 243.

Morton, R. S. (1966). Social aspects of gonorrhoea in the female. *Medical Gynaecology and Sociology,* **1,** 2.

Morton, R. S. (1971). *Sexual Freedom and Venereal Disease.* London: Peter Owen.

Rawlins, D. C. (1967). Drug taking by patients with venereal disease. *British Journal of Venereal Diseases,* **45,** 238.

Schofield, M. (1968). *Sexual Behavior of Young People.* London: Penguin.

Tunnadine, L. P. D. (1970). *Contraception and Sexual Life.* London: Tavistock Publications.

Webster, B. (1970). Venereal disease control in the United States. *British Journal of Venereal Diseases,* **46,** 494.

Wells, B. W. P. (1969). Personality characteristics of V.D. patients. *British Journal of the Society of Clinical Psychology,* **8,** 246.

Wells, B. W. P. (1969). *Social Aspects of Venereal Diseases.* London: British Social Biology Council.

Wells, B. W. P. (1970). Personality study of V.D. patients using the psychoticism, extroversion, neuroticism inventory. *British Journal of Venereal Diseases,* **46,** 498.

Wells, B. W. P. & Schofield, C. B. S. (1970). 'Target' sites for anti-V.D. propaganda. *Health Bulletin. Department of Health for Scotland,* **XXVIII,** 1, 73.

Willcox, R. R. (1965). Venereal disease and immigration. *Practitioner,* **195,** 628.

5. Syphilis

Syphilis is a contagious disease the causal organism of which is the *Treponema pallidum*. Transmission is usually by contagion but it can be passed from a mother to her unborn child. The disease is systemic from the onset, is of great chronicity, its course distinguished by florid manifestations on the one hand and years of complete asymptomatic latency on the other. It is able to simulate many diseases in the fields of medicine and surgery and is transmissible to certain laboratory animals, but as yet *T. pallidum* has not been grown *in vitro*.

TREPONEMA PALLIDUM

Treponema pallidum is a delicate organism of regular narrow spirals measuring about $1 \cdot 0 \ \mu m$ from one crest to the next, but slightly more in depth. Its length varies from 5 to over $20 \ \mu m$ depending on the number of spirals, the breadth being only $0 \cdot 25 \ \mu m$. It can be examined live by darkground microscopy when its movements are seen to consist of: (1) a cork-screw rotation about its long axis, moving forwards and backwards, (2) expansion and contraction of the coils, like a spring, and (3) angulation, when it bends without loss of its regular spiral form, to more than a right angle. It can also be identified by special staining methods in sections of tissue. Silver impregnation has

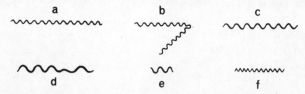

Fig. 6 *T. pallidum* and other spiral organisms. (a) *T. pallidum*. (b) *T. pallidum* showing angling. (c) *T. gracile*. (d) *B. refringens*. (e) *T. balanitidus*. (f) *T. microdentium*. (Reproduced from A. E. W. McLachlan: *Handbook of Diagnosis and Treatment of Venereal Diseases* 3rd edn. Edinburgh: Livingstone.)

been used to demonstrate the organism in the aorta, brain and lymph glands. Recently immunofluorescent techniques have revealed *T. pallidum* in tissues as well as certain body fluids, aqueous humor and cerebrospinal fluid. It divides by transverse fission about once every 30 hours in its active phase, but will not survive outside the body for more than a few hours, being destroyed by heat, drying, antiseptics or soap and water, although it can survive in citrated blood, kept at 4°C for about 3 days.

Treponema pallidum belongs to the treponema group of spirochaetes, some of which cause the treponematoses. This group of diseases includes, in the tropics, yaws, bejel and pinta as well as syphilis, which may be found as an endemic and non-venereal disease in communities living in squalor. Other treponemes are saprophytic, *T. macrodentium* and *T. micro-dentium* in the mouth and *B. refringens* in the genitalia, while a few strains have been grown for many years in laboratories. Among these the Nichols strain has only been maintained in animals and remains pathogenic, while Reiter's strain, which is non-pathogenic, grows on artificial media. *Treponema pallidum* is morphologically indistinguishable from *T. pertenue* and *T. carateum*, respectively, the causal organisms of yaws and pinta, but syphilis can be differentiated from yaws experimentally. Infection of hamsters with *T. pallidum* causes an asymptomatic or latent infection while *T. pertenue* causes marked lesions at the site of scarification.

PATHOLOGY

In acquired syphilis *T. pallidum* invades the body via a mucous membrane, usually genital, or through a skin abrasion. Some of the organisms remain locally and multiply, others disseminate within hours into the reticulo-endothelial system before multiplying. In congenital syphilis there is a blood-borne infection of the foetus via the placenta.

Syphilis is a disease of blood vessels, and the host tissues react to the presence of *T. pallidum* multiplying in the lymphatics and perivascular spaces by: (1) capillary dilatation with swelling and proliferation of the endothelium (when the lumen is closed, causing tissue necrosis distal to the block it is known as obliterative endarteritis). (2) a perivascular infiltration of lymphocytes, plasma cells and giant cells (periarteritis), and later of fibroblasts, with the formation of new blood vessels. Scar tissue is formed, the method of healing of syphilis. The severity and extent of the damage vary according to the state of immunity of the host tissues. In early syphilis the endarteritis causes erosions and ulcers, solitary in the primary stage, but generalized on the mucous membranes and moist skin areas in the secondary. The perivascular infiltration causes the induration of the chancre in primary, and of the papules in secondary syphilis. The macular or roseolar rash of secondary syphilis is caused by the capillary dilatation with endothelial swelling and proliferation. In late syphilis, if there is tissue hypersensitivity to *T. pallidum,* the severity of the obliterative endarteritis may cause considerable tissue destruction (gummas); otherwise the inflammatory changes gradually give way to degenerative ones such as are seen in cardiovascular and neurosyphilis.

IMMUNITY

An initial attack does not give 'complete immunity' as in certain bacterial diseases. Treponemata, re-inoculated into another site during the incubation period of the initial infection, will multiply and produce lesions, but once the primary lesion is established further lesions cannot be produced by subsequent inoculation. The primary lesion of syphilis does not prevent the development of generalized secondary lesions, relapses or late syphilis. Tissues vary in their ability to develop immunity. Some, such as the skin, develop high immunity while others, for example the cornea, have a very low immunity. A florid eruption is said to have a favourable effect on the prognosis. The course of syphilis, after the early stage, depends on the immune response of the host. The majority of patients maintain a level of immunity sufficient to limit the disease to such a low-grade inflammation, leading to fibrosis, as to remain latent. This is not necessarily benign in certain tissues, such as the aorta, where it may lead to aneurysmal dilatation. In other patients tissue hypersensitivity develops to the treponemes, or the products of their destruction. Subsequent invasion of these sensitized tissues causes massive destruction, characteristic of the gumma. Reinfection with *T. pallidum* can occur in cases of late untreated syphilis, either acquired or congenital, or following the successful treatment of an early infection.

It is only in recent years that any amount of research has been directed to the study of the humoral and cellular responses of the host to infection with syphilis. With regard to the immuno-globulins, in primary syphilis initially there is a rise in the level of IgM followed by that of IgG. In secondary syphilis, the level of IgG remains high, that of IgM declines while that of IgA becomes raised. The level of IgG remains raised in the late stages of syphilis while that of IgM approaches normal. To date, neither the presence nor absence of any of these immunoglobulins can be correlated with protection of the host. As far as cell-mediated immunity is concerned the picture is even more obscure. The direct leucocyte migration test, using Reiter protein as an antigen, reveals stimulation of migration in primary and inhibition in late syphilis. This is interpreted as evidence of weak and strong delayed hypersensitivity respectively. In latent syphilis, the finding of stimulation may mean that the infection is of recent origin and of inhibition that it is of some standing. Neither stimulation nor inhibition occurs in secondary syphilis and this may mean failure or suppression of cell-mediated immunity during this stage of infection. However, the ability of lymphocytes of patients with syphilis to undergo blastic trans-formation in response to treponemal antigens is found to be maximum in the secondary stage, the intensity appearing to follow the behaviour of the *Treponema pallidum* immobilization (TPI) test. The cause of this dissociation in secondary syphilis is open to several interpretations which may have to take into account the finding of a factor in the plasma of patients with secondary, but not in those with primary or latent syphilis, which inhibits the phytohaemagglutinin transforma-tion of normal peripheral lymphocytes as well as of their own cells.

AETIOLOGY

Not everyone exposed to syphilis acquires the disease, some appear resistant to infection, and of those who are infected only a proportion develop symptoms, the others are asymptomatic. This might be explained by the size of the infecting dose of organisms, but the later effects of syphilis certainly appear to owe more to the host than the organism. As in botany, it is not so much the seed as the soil which determines whether the plant will thrive or wither.

The infection is usually transmitted by sexual contact and much more rarely by kissing or close bodily contact. The risk of contagion is high during the first 2 to 4 years, after which it is slight. Syphilis can be transmitted by blood transfusion, especially when fresh blood is used, the longest duration of known syphilitic infection in a donor is 7 years, but more frequently the donor is only incubating the disease and the serological tests are negative. In normal circumstances blood banks store citrated blood at 5°C. At this temperature *T. pallidum* disappears in 72 to 96 hours. The risk of an untreated woman infecting her unborn child decreases with time from almost certainty during the first two years of the disease to exceptional rarity after 20 years.

It is well recognized that the course of syphilis is more severe in men than women. Possibly the treponemes can thrive within the stable milieu of men, but find survival more difficult in women, because of their cyclic menstrual hormonal changes. Pregnancy, with its even greater hormonal and chemical variations, has been shown to give an added protection to the parous, especially multiparous, woman against the development of the late lesions of syphilis. Age can be an aetiological factor; a foetus will succumb to the acute infection of syphilis, but this stage is mild in acquired syphilis, the patients only dying from the late results of the disease.

It is said that Negroes are more susceptible to cutaneous, osseous and cardiovascular syphilis than whites who, together with the brown races, have a higher incidence of neurosyphilis. It is uncertain whether this is due to racial or occupational factors, since heavy manual workers are more prone to aneurysm of the aorta than are those in sedentary jobs, while gummas may develop at sites that have been subjected to trauma. Hyperpyrexia will kill treponemes, which die *in vivo* or *in vitro* if kept at 42°C for 1 to 6 hours. Even intercurrent infections, such as malaria, relapsing or undulant fevers, have a beneficial effect on the prognosis of syphilis.

Claims have been made that certain strains of *T. pallidum* show tropism, and tend to cause either cardiovascular or neurosyphilis. The frequency with which both husband and wife suffer from neurosyphilis, also observed in several men infected by one woman, are cited as evidence to support this contention. On the other hand, members of one family, infected from several sources, often suffer from the same type of late syphilis, so the possibility of tropism remains in question.

THE NATURAL COURSE OF SYPHILIS

As already mentioned some patients infected with syphilis fail to develop early clinical manifestations, and it is difficult to estimate what proportion of these will develop late syphilis. The majority of patients attending initially with cardiovascular syphilis have neither a history nor the scars of early syphilis. They aver that, had they noticed any lesions, they would have sought medical advice.

The course of untreated early syphilis is well known from the several studies that have been carried out. The most notable is that carried out by Gjestland from 1949 to 1951 on the so called Boeck-Bruusgaard material. Caesar Boeck was so dissatisfied with the treatment available, that for 20 years (1891 to 1910) in Oslo, he did not treat his patients suffering from primary and secondary syphilis. He simply isolated them in hospital for 1 to 12 months (mean 3·6 months) until their lesions healed, some relapsing on one or more occasions. Gjestland followed up 331 male and 622 female patients and found that the total incidence of late clinical syphilis was 31·1 per cent for males and 26·7 per cent for females. The incidence of the individual types of late syphilis was as follows:

	Males	Females
'Benign' tertiary syphilis	51 (15·4 per cent)	109 (17·5 per cent)
Cardiovascular syphilis	45 (14·2 per cent)	47 (7·6 per cent)
Neurosyphilis	31 (9·4 per cent)	31 (5·0 per cent)

No account was taken of the serological findings in the other patients, but latent syphilis 40 to 60 years after infection carries a very good prognosis, clinical lesions rarely developing, if at all. From this investigation it would appear that, following early clinical syphilis, the majority of patients suffer no late functional effects. Having said that, it must be pointed out that *T. pallidum* has been found persisting in patients following treatment for late syphilis, in one case after over 500 mega units of penicillin, and that some of the patients lacked any serological evidence of syphilis. Treponemes have been found in lymph glands, pharangeal lympoid tissue, aorta, liver, the aqueous humor and cerebrospinal fluid of treated patients, and in some cases rabbits have been infected by those treponemes. From this evidence it appears that *T. pallidum* cannot always be eliminated from the body if treatment is delayed beyond the secondary stage of syphilis, no matter what dosage of penicillin is used.

HISTORY

Syphilis was first recorded and fully described in Europe at the end of the 15th century. It was not described, nor even mentioned, by earlier writers and there is no reason to suppose that those at the turn of the 16th century were any more observant than their forebears, including the great Egyptian, Arabic and Greek writers. Nobody knows the origin of syphilis, although many hold strong views. There are two widely held theories: the Unitarian and the Columbian. According to the former all the present treponematoses have originated from one tropical disease, somewhat similar to present day yaws but in colder climates, where clothing and better cleanliness prevented transmission by bodily contact, it became a venereal disease. Some believe that the disease was spread from Africa through the ancient trade routes and by emigration, and was alluded to in the Book of Deuteronomy although no pathological proof has yet been presented to show its existence in ancient times, or even up to 1494. Others hold that it was not until the 15th century that syphilis was introduced from Africa to Europe by slaves and traders operating on the West coast of Africa. According to the Columbian theory, syphilis was imported to Europe in 1493 by the crews of Christopher Columbus's expedition which reached the West Indies in 1492. Some of the crew members are said to have acquired syphilis from the local women and to have developed a rash 'Indian Measles', on the voyage home to Palos in Spain, where they were paid off. Later some of them are supposed to have been mercenary soldiers in the army of Charles VIII of France at the siege of Naples. After the city was conquered in 1494 an epidemic of syphilis broke out which so weakened the soldiers that the French army had to be disbanded. The mercenaries were thus scattered throughout Europe taking the infection with them. The French army called the disease the 'Neopolitan' or 'Italian' disease, the Italians called it the 'French' disease. Syphilis reached France, Germany and Switzerland in 1495; the Netherlands and Greece in 1496; England and Scotland in 1497; Hungary and Russia in 1499. It is said to have been exported from Europe by Vasco da Gama's sailors and to have reached India in 1498 and China in 1505.

The name, syphilis, was coined by Frascatorius of Verona for the anti-hero of his popular and famous poem, 'Syphilis, sive Morbus Gallicus', which was published in 1530. Thenceforward the disease was known as syphilis, although initially it was not appreciated that the disease was sexually transmitted. In the 16th century Paracelsus recognized its congenital character, Ambroise Paré that it caused aortic aneurysms and Ulrich von Hutton recommended treatment with guiaicum and mercury. Sydenham used mercury by inunction in the 17th century and, although it could be very toxic and cures were uncertain, it remained the treatment of choice for the next two centuries or more. By the 18th century it was realized that syphilis and gonorrhoea were sexually transmitted, but they had not been differentiated. In his famous experiment John Hunter inoculated himself with pus from a man suffering from gonorrhoea. Unfortunately, the patient also had syphilis and Hunter developed both syphilis and gonorrhoea. He, and others, concluded that the diseases were one and the same. Owing to Hunter's regrettable mistake it was not until 1839 that the difference was established by Philip Ricord. The causal organism of gonorrhoea, *Neisseria gonorrhoeae*, was not discovered until 1879 by Albert Neisser and that of syphilis, *Treponema pallidum*, in 1905 by Schaudinn and Hoffman, the latter by darkground microscopy. The Wassermann reaction was developed by Wassermann, Neisser and Bruck in 1906, shortly after the publication of the Bordet and Gengou phenomenon of complement fixation. The next year Ehrlich, who had been developing organic arsenical compounds, discovered in his 606th experiment his 'magic-bullets' arsphenamine, which he called Salvarsan or '606'. This intravenous chemotherapeutic agent was toxic and unstable, but in his 914th experiment Ehrlich produced neoarsphenamine which was easier to inject and less toxic. In 1917, Wagner-Jauregg first used malaria to produce a fever in the treatment of neurosyphilis. Sazerac and Levaditi, in 1921, introduced bismuth which could be given by intramuscular injections, and this 'rug, together with neoarsphenamine intravenously, was the standard treatment for syphilis until penicillin became available. Mahoney, Arnold and Harris were the first, in 1943, to treat syphilis with penicillin. Such is its efficiency and relative lack of toxicity that it remains the drug of choice in every stage of syphilis.

The most recent discoveries have all been in the development of specific serological tests for syphilis. In 1949 Nelson and Mayer introduced the *Treponema pallidum* immobilization (TPI) Test which, owing to the complexity of the techniques required, could only be carried out in a few laboratories. Later, Deacon, Falcone and Harris, in 1957, described a fluorescent treponemal antibody (FTA) test which could be done in any serological laboratory but which was relatively insensitive. In 1964, Hunter, Deacon and Meyer developed a method of absorbing out the non-specific antigens and the resulting test, the absorbed fluorescent treponemal antibody (FTA-ABS) test is now the most specific and sensitive serological test in current use. The *Treponema pallidum* haemagglutinization assay (TPHA) test was originally described by Rathlev in 1965. It has since been developed and using an automated microtechnique (AMHA-TP test) is the first specific test suitable for screening purposes.

EPIDEMIOLOGY

The incidence of syphilis has been declining in Europe and North America since about 1860. Earle Moore believed this to be due to improved social conditions rather than to treatment, and that transitory increases could be accounted for by wars and

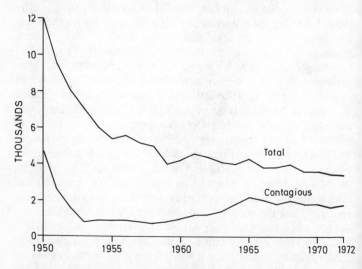

Fig. 7 Syphilis in Britain 1950-1972; total and contagious cases.

migrations. In Britain the incidence of late syphilis did not start to decline until the early 1950s, but the death rate for neurosyphilis has been falling since the 1930s and that for aneurysms of the aorta since the 1940s. The incidence of deaths due to congenital syphilis in the first year of life has fallen since the turn of the 20th century to almost zero over the past 10 years.

The incidence of early syphilis in Britain fell from the post-war peak in 1946 until the early 1950s. This may have been due, in part, to the increasing amount of penicillin used at that time for so many other conditions. With the development of the broad-spectrum antibiotics, less effective in the treatment of syphilis, penicillin is not now so widely used. During the late 1950s the number of new cases remained fairly steady, but from 1959 rose sharply until 1965, since when the incidence has dropped a little and remained fairly steady.

FURTHER READING

Deacon, W. E., Falcone, V. H. & Harris, A. (1957). Fluorescent test for treponemal antibodies. *Proceedings of the Society for Experimental Biology and Medicine,* **96,** 477.

Frascatoro, G. *Syphilis or the French Disease.* With translation notes and appendix by Heneage Wynne-Finch (1935). London: Heinemann.

Fulford, K. W. M. & Brostoff, J. (1972). Leucocyte migration and cell mediated immunity in syphilis. *British Journal of Venereal Diseases,* **48,** 483.

Gestland, T. (1955). The Oslo study of untreated syphilis. An epidemiological investigation of the natural course of the syphilitic infection based upon the re-study of the Boeck Bruusgaard material. *Acta dermato-venereologica (Stockholm),* **35,** Suppl. 34.

Hunter, E. F., Deacon, W. E. & Myer, P. E. (1964). An improved FTA test for syphilis, the absorption procedure (FTA-ABS). *Public Health Reports (Washington),* 79, 410.

McLachlan, A. E. W. (1947). *Handbook of Diagnosis and Treatment of Venereal Diseases,* 3rd edn. Edinburgh: Livingstone.

Morton, R. S. & Harris, R. J. W. (1974). *Recent Advances in Sexually Transmitted Diseases,* Edinburgh and London: Churchill Livingstone.

Ovcinnikov, N. M. & Delectorskij, V. V. (1968). Further studies of ultrathin sections of *Treponema pallidum* under the electron microscope. *British Journal of Venereal Diseases,* **44,** 1.

Smith, J. L. (1969). *Spirochetes in Late Seronegative Syphilis, Penicillin Notwithstanding.* Springfield, Illinois: Thomas.

Stokes, J. H., Beerman, H. & Ingraham, N. R. (1945). *Modern Clinical Syphilology,* 3rd edn. Philadelphia: Saunders.

Treponematosis Research (1970). *WHO Technical Report Series.* Geneva, No. 455.

Wright, D. J. M. & Grimble, A. S. (1974). Why is the infectious stage of syphilis prolonged? *British Journal of Venereal Diseases*, **50**, 45.

Yobs, A. R., Clark, J. W., Mothershed, S. E., Bullard, J. C. & Attley, C. W. (1968). Further observations on the persistence of *Treponema pallidum*. *British Journal of Venereal Diseases*, **44**, 111.

6. Serological Tests for Syphilis and Their Interpretation

Correct use of the serological tests for syphilis now available should enable the clinician to eliminate or diagnose with certainty syphilis, or at least a treponematosis, and give an accurate prognosis. It is therefore essential for him to have the collaboration of a serologist, who requires an adequate history with each specimen of blood, to know whether screening, diagnostic or prognostic tests are required. There are two types of serological tests: (1) Non-specific screening or standard tests (STS), which test for the presence of reagin, and (2) tests for specific antitreponemal antibodies.

Laboratories which receive relatively few specimens may test them only once a week, or less frequently, with a consequent delay in reporting; this is to the disadvantage of clinicians and patients, while the paucity of positive results tends to detract from job-satisfaction within the laboratory. Furthermore, a lack of positive control sera may, on occasion, cause difficulties in the interpretation of results.

A better service can be provided by a few laboratories testing large numbers of sera, preferably using the automated techniques now available. No other laboratory test is carried out on so large a scale, and for such a meagre yield of positive results, as are the serological tests for syphilis. This is certainly so as far as the screening of antenatal patients and blood donors is concerned. Nevertheless, the importance of this work cannot be overemphasized and, in many countries, serological tests for syphilis are required by law to be carried out in certain circumstances.

Automation of flocculation and complement fixation tests is usually by means of a continuous flow system, which carries with it the risk that a strongly positive specimen may trail behind it contaminants which could affect a succeeding negative specimen and give a false positive result. Automation of the haemagglutination assay test is by the more costly technique of discrete analysis, which obviates the problem of contamination as each specimen is segregated in its own container throughout, the various reagents being added to it during the course of the test.

Two bottlenecks remain for all the automated tests. Serum must be separated from the blood samples received by the laboratory and the 'read-outs' on paper of the flocculation and complement fixation tests, or the results of the haemagglutination test, have to be scrutinized and transcribed to written reports by an experienced observer. Nevertheless, automation can take much of the drudgery out of syphilis serology and certainly speeds up the reporting of accurate results to the clinician.

NON-SPECIFIC SEROLOGICAL TESTS

Reagin. (Not to be confused with the term reagin as used by immunologists, the skin sensitizing antibody which belongs to the 1gE class of immunoglobulins.) The serum of a patient suffering from syphilis contains an excess of reagin, part of the gamma-globulin fraction of serum, usually by about the fifth week after infection, but it may not be detectable until the thirteenth. It is not specific for syphilis or even the treponematoses, being present in other diseases and conditions. Reagin will combine with colloidal suspensions of tissue lipids to form visible clumps or floccules, especially if the mixture is shaken. Another property of this reagin-lipid complex is its ability to 'fix', or combine with, complement. (Complement is a non-specific component of normal serum which can lyse, or destroy, an antigen once that antigen has been sensitized by contact with an immune body. Guinea-pig serum, which is rich in complement is normally used.)

On the basis of these properties two types of STS have been developed: flocculation tests and complement fixation tests. The active principle in the colloidal extracts of tissue lipids is cardiolipin, a phospholipid found in mammalian heart muscle, which, when mixed with lecithin and cholesterol in suitable proportions, forms a sensitive antigen for the detection of reagin.

Flocculation tests

Over the years many flocculation tests have been developed, such as the Kahn, Kline, Meinicke, Price and the Venereal Disease Research Laboratory (VDRL) Test, and it is the latter which has found most favour, being relatively reliable, simple to perform either as a tube test or, as is more usual, as a slide test, while the results are reproducible throughout the world.

VDRL slide test

Cardiolipin antigen suspension is added to inactivated serum on a slide which is rotated, to ensure mixing, for 4 minutes and then examined under a low-power (X 100) microscope to detect floccules of antigen particles if the result is positive. (Inactivation is accomplished by heating serum at 56°C for 30 minutes, the purpose being to abolish non-specific effects. By this means also naturally occuring complement in the patient's serum is inactivated, a point of importance in complement fixation tests but not in the VDRL test, because complement plays no part in flocculation.) By serially diluting the serum in normal saline a quantitative result can be obtained. Sometimes, however, sera containing large amounts of antibody give false-negative results when tested undiluted, or in low dilutions, but when retested at higher dilution show strong flocculation. This is called a prozone reaction, a well-known phenomenon which occasionally occurs in all flocculation tests but not with complement fixation tests.

Automated reagin test (ART)

The ART is the VDRL test adapted for automation. The antigen consists of cardiolipin absorbed onto very fine particles of charcoal suspended in buffered saline and the test is carried out at room temperature. The equipment consists of an autoanalyser having in its circuit reaction, mixing and settling coils and, at the end, a moving ribbon of filter paper for the 'read out'. It takes 16 minutes for a sample to traverse the system, but once running the machine can perform 100 tests per hour. The sera to be tested, and with each run known positive and negative control sera, are placed in 36 of the 40 cups of the sampler turntable. Each tenth cup contains a vegetable dye solution to act as markers. A sampling probe draws up the required volume of serum or dye, by suction from a vacuum pump, into the system's narrow, transparent plastic tubing. Each sample is followed by an air bubble (air-break), then saline (three times the volume of the sample), then another air-break and then a succeeding sample. Consecutive samples are thus separated by a saline wash sandwiched between two air-breaks. Progress of these segments through the system is aided by a peristaltic pump, a revolving cam which squeezes the tubing, 'milking' its contents onwards.

To each segment of serum, saline or dye is added an amount of ART antigen suspension (one-third the volume of the serum) by means of a T-junction just before the mixtures enter the reaction coils. These are spiral glass coils wound closely together around a horizontal axis which cause the continuous tumbling and thorough mixing of the serum and antigen suspension over a period of eight minutes. More saline is added to each segment via another T-junction and the diluted mixtures pass through a shorter set of coils in which the particulate matter is dispersed in preparation for the 'settling' stage of the test. This is accomplished in a coil of one and a half loops round a circle of much wider diameter than the previous coils and wound around a vertical axis. As the mixtures pass slowly round this relatively long settling coil there is ample time for the particles to fall out of suspension and form a deposit on the bottom of the moving fluid segments. Surplus clear supernatant fluid and the air bubbles are aspirated via a third T-junction into a waste container, leaving the concentrated deposit to travel onward to a dispensing microprobe. This is a small-bore metal tube with its smooth, flat, open end resting lightly on a moving ribbon of filter paper beneath which is a wider suction tube leading to the waste container.

As each specimen emerges from the metal tube, ART antigens are deposited onto the filter paper to form a linear mark, the excess fluid being sucked through the paper and discarded. If the serum has not reacted with the antigen suspension, the linear mark is an even, very faint, grey smudge and the result is read as negative. If the serum has caused the antigen to flocculate, the linear mark has a 'black-peppered' appearance, the stronger the reaction the more marked the visible specks which are clumps of carbon/antigen particles, indicating a positive result. The concentration of antigen suspension in the saline segments is so small that smudge formed is almost invisible. The reading of results is facilitated by these virtual blank spaces between the deposits left by the serum samples. Identification of the results of individual sera is made easier by the dye, present in every tenth specimen. As a precaution, whenever a sample giving a strong positive reaction is followed by one regarded as positive, the latter should be retested in case it might be a 'carry-over' fallacy, the sample possibly having been contaminated by its predecessor through the system.

Sera giving positive results are retested to titre by serial dilution in successive cups on the sampler turntable, so that the results may be reported quantitatively. This should also be done whenever a negative result is obtained with neat serum, in the face of a clinical or historical suspicion of syphilis, in case of a prozone reaction.

Complement fixation tests

The Wassermann reaction (WR) was the first of the complement fixation tests to be used in the diagnosis of syphilis. Many variations have been developed in the search for better selectivity with sufficient sensitivity and adequate reproducibility. The cardiolipin Wassermann reaction (CWR) is the test now most commonly used, being the most sensitive and reproducible, yet selective because the reagents are prepared from chemically pure substances.

Cardiolipin Wassermann Reaction (CWR)

Inactivated serum, cardiolipin antigen and complement are mixed together in a tube and with a control tube, containing only serum and complement, are incubated at 37°C for an hour; complement is fixed by the serum-antigen mixture if reagin is present, but remains free if not. To test for the presence or absence of free complement a haemolytic or 'indicator system' is added to both tubes which are incubated at 37°C for a further half hour. The haemolytic system consists of amboceptor and washed sheep red-cells, which are haemolysed in the presence of free complement. (Amboceptor is an immune body present in rabbit anti-serum to sheep red cells. It is prepared by repeatedly injecting a rabbit with sheep red cells.) Known positive and negative sera are included with each batch of sera tested. Lack of haemolysis indicates complement fixation and the presence of reagin. This is reported as a positive reaction. Partial haemolysis, due to the presence of only a small amount of reagin, is reported as 'weak positive' or 'doubtful'. Complete haemolysis is reported as negative. There should be complete haemolysis in the control tube, if not the serum must be reported as anti-complementary, and a further specimen of the patient's serum tested later.

False-positive reactions to non-specific tests

In the absence of reagin, false-positive reactions can be reported due to human errors and the use of faulty reagents. Reagin can also be present in health, in diseases other than syphilis and in the other treponematoses.

Human and technical errors. Mistakes can occur at any point from the moment blood is collected from the patient to the time when the laboratory report is entered in the case notes. Incorrect labelling, bacteriological contamination of the specimen, undue delay and shaking while in transport, faulty laboratory equipment and reagents, errors in reading, recording and typing the results, or in transcribing them to case notes, all contribute to the number of false-positive results recorded. It is important therefore never to rely on the result of one test alone, nor even on the results of several tests carried out on a single specimen, without definite clinical evidence of syphilis.

In health. During pregnancy some normal non-syphilitic women produce an excess of reagin; in fact only between 10 and 20 per cent of positive ante-natal STS are confirmed by the specific tests. In addition a few healthy people, especially the elderly, are found to have an excess of reagin in the absence of disease.

Biological false-positive (BFP) reactions. These can occur in both acute and chronic forms. An acute or transient BFP reaction may occur in the course of almost any fever, but particularly with virus pneumonia, infectious mononucleosis, active pulmonary tuberculosis, leptospirosis and vaccinia, and in the tropics in particular, with malaria, typhus and filariasis. BFP reactions are considered to be chronic when of over 6 months duration and are associated with chronic conditions such as systemic lupus erythematosus, rheumatoid arthritis, cirrhosis of the liver, psoriasis and in the tropics with leprosy. Recently an association has been confirmed with drug addiction.

Other treponematoses. The tropical and sub-tropical diseases, yaws, bejel and pinta, are all caused by treponemas closely related to *Treponema pallidum.* Patients suffering from them have reagin in their sera and as the specific serological tests cannot distinguish syphilis from the other treponematoses, positive STS results are therefore not false. This must be borne in mind when interpreting positive results on patients born and brought up in areas where one of these diseases has been prevalent.

False-negative reactions to non-specific tests

Human and technical errors. Whenever, owing to human error, a false-positive result has been reported, then it is possible that a false-negative report will have been issued on serum containing an excess of reagin, and this missed diagnosis can be even more dangerous. Technical errors rarely cause false-negative reactions, while other noted causes, pregnancy, alcohol or an anaesthetic, must be very rare indeed. The only way to avoid the possible consequences of any false reaction is to ensure that the results of one specimen are always confirmed by another.

SPECIFIC SEROLOGICAL TESTS

The specific serological tests use treponemal antigens which are obtained either from cultivable non-pathogenic treponemes or by using *T. pallidum* itself as an antigen. None of these tests can differentiate between the various treponematoses, but a positive result is diagnostic of syphilis in patients born outside those areas where the tropical varieties are prevalent.

Tests using antigens from cultivable treponemes

Reiter protein complement fixation test (RPCFT)

This is a complement fixation test using a protein antigen prepared by the disruption of washed Reiter's treponemes, the protein being precipitated by ammonium sulphate. Reiter's treponemes, although originally isolated from a genital lesion, are non-pathogenic for rabbits and man, have been grown *in vitro* for many years and are thought to be more closely related to *B. refringens* than to *T. pallidum,* with which, however, they do share common antigens.

False-positive reactions. Occasional false-positive reactions are due to an antibody against lipopolysaccharide antigens present in the protein extract. The antibody detected by the RPCFT is distinct from that detected by reagin tests and differs from that causing false-positive reactions with reagin. The likelihood of their co-existence in one patient is small.

False-negative reactions. The sensitivity of the RPCFT is such that it can detect a syphilitic infection at an early stage but when the disease is of many years' duration, and especially in a treated case, it is not as sensitive as the other specific tests.

Automated RPCFT

The autoanalyser for complement fixation tests differs from that used for the ART in that it has two sets of reaction coils and the results are read by means of a flow cell rather than on a moving ribbon of filter paper. Each sample takes 40 minutes to traverse the system and the throughput is 80 samples per hour.

The sampling procedure is similar to that of the ART except that the dye is not used. At the first T-junction, the required volume of correctly proportioned antigen/complement mixture is added to each serum sample and saline wash, which then proceeds to the first set of reaction coils. Non-specific antigen can be used but Reiter protein is to be preferred and, as with all CFTs, complement must be titrated before the start of each run but this can be done by the machine.

The reaction coils are completely immersed in a water bath kept at 37°C and each segment takes about 18 minutes to traverse them. It is during this period that complement fixation, if it is going to occur, takes place. After this the haemolytic system is added via another T-junction and, still in the water bath, the segments proceed through a second set of reaction coils, taking about 16 minutes to do so. In these, if complement has not been fixed in the first set, haemolysis occurs. As in the ART, the segments then pass another T-junction, where saline diluent is added, through a mixing coil and, having emerged from the water bath, the air bubbles are aspirated off before the segments proceed, prior to disposal, through the sensing part of the flow cell. This consists of a short length of precision-made glass tubing lying athwart the light path of a photoelectric cell. Interruption or scatter of the light beam alters the otherwise constant electric current generated by the photo-cell. These changes are detected by a sensitive galvanometer and traced on a moving band of ruled paper by means of a stylograph at the end of a delicately counterbalanced pivoted arm, to which the galvanometer is linked. If intact red blood cells are deposited on the bottom of a segment of fluid, because the complement has been fixed in the first set of reaction coils, they will interrupt or scatter the light beam and cause such a variation in current that a sharp peak is recorded on the tracing. This is reported as a positive result. The higher the peak, the more strongly positive the result, thus adding a quantitative element to the other advantages of this automated test. The faint optical density of non reactive specimens and of the saline rinses, due to the serum or saline, complement, antigen and the haemoglobin from the lysed cells, is only sufficient to cause a minor 'hump' in the tracing, but the contrast between this and the sharp peak of a positive result is very obvious. As with the ART quantitative results can be obtained by the serial dilution of the serum in consecutive cups on the sampler turntable.

Tests using Treponema pallidum as an antigen

Treponema pallidum immobilization (TPI) test

The TPI test was the first one in which *T. pallidum* was used as an antigen. It was introduced by Nelson and Mayer in 1949, after they had developed a medium in which *T. pallidum* survived and remained motile for several days, although they did not multiply. They found that inactivated serum from patients suffering from syphilis, in the presence of complement, immobilized virulent *T. pallidum* when they were incubated together at 35°C for 18 hours. The mixture is examined by darkground microscopy and if 50 per cent or more treponemes are immobilized the test is reported positive, if 20 per cent or less the test is negative and results in between are regarded as doubtful. The virulent treponemes required for the test are obtained from rabbit testes with syphilitic orchitis, the supply of organisms being perpetuated by serial passage of infected material intra-testicularly from one rabbit to another. The technique of the test is very complicated and few laboratories are equipped to perform it.

Immobilizing antibody is distinct from antibodies detected by reagin tests as well as from group anti-treponemal antibody detected by the RPCFT. The TPI test is the last to become positive in early syphilis, and if treatment is given early enough will not become positive. It is positive in all cases of established secondary and latent syphilis, and unfortunately usually remains so in the majority of patients despite adequate treatment. It is therefore quite useless for assessing prognosis, as the persistence of a positive result in the absence of clinical evidence of continued disease activity is not an indication for further therapy.

False-negative reactions. *Treponema pallidum* is very sensitive to penicillin, and false-negative results may occur if the patient has been treated with penicillin or any other treponemicidal drug recently.

Fluorescent treponemal antibody tests

These tests are carried out by the indirect method. In the first stage the patient's serum is applied to a film of *T. pallidum* fixed on a slide. If anti-treponemal antibody is present in the serum it will unite with the treponemal antigen. In the second stage anti-human globulin, conjugated with fluorescein isothiocyanate, is added and this in turn unites with the antibody attached to the treponemes, which fluoresce when examined by darkground microscopy with an ultraviolet light source. There is no fluorescence unless there is antibody in the serum. The early fluorescent tests gave false-positive reactions because many sera contain antibodies, in low titre, to group-antigens found in other treponemes, mainly commensals in the mouth and genitalia. To minimize the risk of these false-positive reactions sera were tested at a dilution of one part in 200 (FTA–200). This test, although specific for *T. pallidum,* was relatively insensitive.

Absorbed fluorescent treponemal antibody (FTA-ABS) test

In this test group-reactive antibodies are absorbed out of the serum by a sorbent. (Sorbent consists of intact or disintegrated Reiter's treponemes.) This makes it possible to perform the test on sera diluted only one part in five, thus enhancing its sensitivity without impairing its specificity. The FTA-ABS test is as specific and more sensitive than the TPI, and all the other serological tests, in every stage of syphilis. It is usually the first to become positive in untreated primary syphilis and, like the TPI test, it reverts to negative if treatment is given early in the disease, but not very often if it is delayed until the later stages, although a modification of the test, the FTA-IgM, does revert to negative within a reasonable time of treatment in early and late syphilis.

False-positive reactions. Sera containing abnormal globulins and anti-nuclear factor, or more rarely rheumatoid factor, very occasionally give rise to false-positive reactions. In the absence of syphilis, further absorption with calf thymus DNA may remove these borderline reactions.

Treponema pallidum haemagglutination assay (TPHA) test

An indirect haemagglutination technique is used in which initially the antigen, *T. pallida* disrupted by sonication, is absorbed onto 'tanned' red blood cells, thus sensitizing them. Rathlev used sheep erythrocytes but more recently those from fowls have been preferred. The reagent is prepared by incubating together, for 30 minutes at 37°C, a suspension of the tanned red blood cells and the treponemal antigen, diluted to the required titre. After washing thoroughly in saline the sensitized cells are resuspended in saline containing 1·5 per cent rabbit serum if for immediate use or preserved by freeze-drying (lyophilisation). The reagent must be used within a short time of reconstitution.

For the actual test measured volumes of sensitized cells and of diluted, inactivated serum from the patient are pipetted into the well of an agglutination tray. After shaking, to ensure thorough mixing, the tray is left undisturbed at room temperature or at 37°C for 30 to 45 minutes to allow the cells to settle. If, on examination, the cells have settled into a compact round 'button' with a smooth entire edge then agglutination has not taken place and the result is read as negative. However, if the cells are spread out in a granular deposit on the bottom of the well, because they were agglutinated before settling, then the result is read as positive.

The TPHA test is an easy one to perform even in peripheral laboratories and the results are reproducible. With serial dilution of individual sera quantitative results can be obtained and the test can be adopted to suit automated techniques, notably that using only minute quantities of sera and reagent, the automated microhaemagglutination (T. pallidum) [AMHA(TP)] test, the best screening test for treponematoses to date.

The sensitivity and specificity of the TPHA test compare favourably with those of the TPI and FTA-ABS tests. It is positive in between 60 to 70 per cent of cases of primary syphilis and thereafter positive in almost all untreated cases. Once positive, the test often remains so for many years, its persistance in this respect outlasting even the TPI test.

False-positive reactions. Very occasionally false positive results have been reported, usually in association with chronic BFP reactions.

Recommended usage of serological tests

Screening tests. Ideally, automated tests should be used whenever large numbers of sera have to be screened. The most sensitive and selective automated one is the AMHA(TP) test, the use of which eliminates the problem of BFP reactions. When the special equipment for that test is not available, and when a negative result is generally expected, then the automated reagin (AR) test and an automated RPCF test should be carried out. In default of automated tests, then a VDRL slide test and a RPCFT should suffice. If both are reported negative the chance of missing syphilis is slight, and then only in its very late stages when, without clinical signs, treatment is rarely warranted. If the result of the RPCFT is anti-complementary the test should be repeated on a fresh specimen of serum. If the results of either is positive or doubtful or if there is anything clinically suspicious, then specific tests should be carried out.

Diagnostic tests. Whenever syphilis is suspected or either of the screening tests show some reaction a specific test should be carried out together with a quantitative VDRL test, if it was positive with neat serum. When the results are in agreement there is no need for further serological investigation, but if they are divergent then a TPI test should be done. It is also wise to carry out the FTA-ABS test, when, in the absence of clinical signs, a patient is suspected of having syphilis of only a few weeks' duration.

Prognostic tests. Once a patient has been diagnosed and treated for syphilis, or any treponematosis, it is essential for the clinician to be able to judge the prognosis of the disease. This is best done by observing the results of serial quantitative VDRL tests, carried out over a period of time; if the titre falls the prognosis is satisfactory, but if it rises again then treatment has failed.

Serological diagnosis of syphilis in neonates. All maternal antibodies, except IgM antibodies, cross the placenta and enter the foetal circulation where they can attain titres identical with those in the mother's blood. This applies both to reagin and to specific antibodies, but not to anti-treponemal antibodies, because they are part of the IgM fraction of globulin, and it applies whether or not the mother has received adequate treatment for syphilis. Carefully collected cord blood, not squeezed out, is only worth testing when the mother has received no treatment, or has been inadequately treated; otherwise it is not only useless, merely demonstrating the passive transfer of antibodies across the placenta, but can be dangerous if the positive results from the baby are taken as an indication of infection with syphilis. The prime use of cord blood is for the carrying out of a FTA-IgM test, which if positive shows that the baby is producing antibody. On occasions cord blood may be of use for the quantitative VDRL test; if it gives a positive result at a higher titre than the mother's blood, the baby probably has syphilis.

Serological elimination of syphilis in neonates. When a baby has no clinical evidence of syphilis serial RPCFT, CWR and quantitative VDRL tests carried out during the first three, or more, months of life will show a fall in titre to negativity within two months for the CWR and VDRL test, the RPCFT sometimes taking longer. If the baby has been infected then the titre will rise.

Interpretation of serological results

While the amounts of the individual antibodies produced varies from person to person there is some consistency in the time of appearance of reagin and of the antibodies detected by the specific tests, although there is no set pattern to the order of their disappearance.

Untreated contagious syphilis. The FTA-ABS test is often found positive when the syphilitic infection is 3 weeks old, and, during the next week the VDRL test, CWR and RPCFT become positive, usually in that order, but often more or less simultaneously. TPHA antibody does not appear in significant amounts until the primary stage is well established. Thereafter, it increases at a steady rate for some months, so that in untreated contagious syphilis, the TPHA titre is a good guide to the duration of infection. The TPI test is the last to become positive, usually at about the sixth week, but it may not become positive until secondary syphilis has become established.

Treated contagious syphilis. During the first week or two of treatment some tests, initially negative, may become positive and the titres of those already positive may rise. Starting treatment does not immediately stop the production of reagin or specific antibody. The serological tests usually revert to negative between 3 and 6 months after treatment. The CWR is often the first in this respect, followed by either the RPCFT or VDRL test in primary syphilis; in secondary syphilis the RPCFT becomes negative before the VDRL test; the FTA-IgM test reverts to negative after 6 to 9 months but the FTA-ABS and TPI tests remain positive for many years in most cases. Serological relapse occurs when, after the titre has dropped even to negativity, it starts to rise again and, unless further treatment is given, clinical relapse may follow.

Untreated late syphilis. Owing to the widespread use of the broad-spectrum antibiotics, patients with late syphilis are rarely untreated at the time of diagnosis; most of them will have received varying amounts of antibiotics in the preceding years. This can make the serological diagnosis very difficult. The VDRL test is usually positive, although the titre varies considerably.

Sometimes the CWR is negative, as is the RPCFT, which may become positive with treatment. The FTA-ABS and TPHA tests are always positive and the TPI test usually so, but it may be negative in long-standing cases such as burnt out tabes dorsalis and late congenital syphilis. On a few occasions the reagin tests will be negative and the RPCFT positive or the reagin tests and the RPCFT all negative and the FTA-ABS test positive. Whether these results call for treatment is a decision best left to the specialist.

Treated late syphilis. Serological reversal of any of the tests may take a long time, with a slow and fluctuating drop in titre. The CWR is often the first to revert, followed by either the RPCFT or VDRL test. In many patients' sera, one test will be negative and another positive on one occasion, but the position reversed at a later date, and this can go on for years. The FTA-IgM test reverts to negative in 1 to 2 years after treatment. Persistence of a positive FTA-IgM test in any stage of treated syphilis may reflect the persistence of treponemes. The FTA-ABS, TPHA and the TPI tests usually remain positive for a very long time indeed and the vast majority of patients suffer no ill. A few, however, have been found to harbour treponeme-like organisms in the aqueous humor, lymph glands, liver, aorta and cerebrospinal fluid. In a few cases the organisms have been proved to be virulent *T. pallidum* by successful animal inoculation. These patients had been treated, apparently adequately, for latent or late syphilis, and in some cases the FTA-ABS and TPI tests were repeatedly reported negative. It is to be regretted that we do not have any test that will tell us when the last *T. pallidum* has been eliminated from the body.

FURTHER READING

Alford, C. A., Polt, S. S., Cassidy, G. E., Straumfjord, J. V. & Remington, J. S. (1969). Gamma-m-fluorescent treponemal antibody in the diagnosis of congenital syphilis. *New England Journal of Medicine,* **280,** 1086.

Ass. Clin. Path. Broadsheet, No. 41. Serological notes for Syphilis. (Whitechapel WR and RPCFT techniques, VDRL).

Dunlop, E. M. C. (1972). Persistance of treponemes after treatment. *British Medical Journal,* **2,** 577.

Hunter, E. F., Norins, L. C., Falcone, V. H. & Stout, G. W. (1968). The fluorescent treponemal antibody-absorbtion (FTA-ABS) test. Development, use and present status. *Bulletin of the World Health Organization,* **39,** 873.

Johnston, N. A. & Wilkinson, A. E. (1968). Absorbed fluorescent antibody (FTA-ABS) test: a comparison with the FTA-200 and TPI tests on 1056 problem sera. *British Journal of Venereal Diseases*, 44, 287.

Johnston, N. A. (1972). Neonatal congenital syphilis. Diagnosis by the absorbed fluorescent treponemal antibody (IgM) test. *British Journal of Venereal Diseases*, 48, 465.

Johnston, N. A. (1972). Treponema pallidum haemagglutination test for syphilis. Evaluation of a modified micro-method. *British Journal of Venereal Diseases*, 48, 474.

Morton, R. S. & Harris, R. J. W. (1974). *Recent Advances in Sexually Transmitted Diseases*. Edinburgh and London: Churchill Livingstone.

O'Neill, P. & Nicol, C. S. (1972). IgM class antitreponemal antibody in treated and untreated syphilis. *British Journal of Venereal Diseases*, 48, 460.

O'Neill, P., Warner, R. W. & Nichol, C. S. (1973). Treponema pallidum haemagglutination assay in the routine serodiagnosis of treponemal disease. *British Journal of Venereal Diseases*, 49, 427.

Portnoy, J. (1965). A note on the performance of modifications of the rapid plasma reagin (RPR) card test for syphilis, for use in large scale testing. *The Public Health Laboratory*, 23, 43.

Schofield, C. B. S. (1973). Serological tests for syphilis in pregnancy. False and missed positive reactions. *British Journal of Venereal Diseases*, 49, 420.

Smith, J. L. (1969). *Spirochetes in Late Seronegative Syphilis, Penicillin Notwithstanding*. Springfield, Illinois: Thomas.

United States Public Health Service (1969). *Manual of Serologic Tests for Syphilis*. U.S. Department of Health Education and Welfare, Publ. No. 411.

Venereal Disease Research Laboratory, Atlanta. (1970). *Automated qualitative and quantitative micro-haemagglutiantion assay for Treponema pallidum antibodies (AMHA-Tp)*. Provisional technique. Modified October 20, 1970.

Wilkinson, A. E. (1970). The positive Wassermann reaction; investigations and interpretation. *British Journal of Hospital Medicine*, 4, 47.

7. Early Contagious Syphilis

The clinical course of untreated syphilis can vary considerably between one patient and another, even in the early stages which principally affect tissues of ectodermal origin. Treponemes abound but, as there is no tissue hypersensitivity, residual damage is minimal. The primary sore, or chancre, commonly has an incubation period of 3 to 4 weeks, but this can vary from 9 days to 3 months; untreated it may take 2 months or more to heal. The generalized rash of secondary syphilis appears at least 6 weeks after infection, usually at about 2 months (but can be delayed up to a year), over 25 per cent of patients with secondary syphilis still having a primary sore. The rash takes several weeks to develop, and is usually most florid 3 to 4 months after infection. After a further period of weeks or months the rash begins to fade, either partially, leaving a few scattered nodules, or completely so that at the end of the first year all the lesions may have disappeared. The disease is now in the stage of early latency. Muco-cutaneous relapses, however, can occur during the second year, and much more rarely beyond that for 2 years, after which no further contagious lesions develop. All early lesions are potentially contagious but the moist ones are invariably and dangerously so, *T. pallidum* abounding in the serous exudates.

PRIMARY SYPHILIS

As the disease is systemic from the outset it is not surprising that some patients have constitutional disturbances to a greater or lesser degree. Headache, pyrexia, pains in the joints, malaise and anaemia occur in about 25 per cent of patients, especially in women.

The Chancre

The primary sore develops at the site of inoculation. Starting as a macule, a spot that can be seen but not felt, it is usually dull-red in colour but may appear as a 'silver spot', often alleged by patients to be a cigarette burn. The macule develops into a papule, which can be both seen and felt. The surface becomes eroded giving rise to an ulcer about 1·0 cm in diameter.

Characteristics of the chancre. Certain clinical findings are common to the majority of primary sores: (1) The sore is usually solitary, but two 'kissing' lesions may be found opposite one another when the mucous membranes are in apposition, as in the subpreputial sac or between the labia. (2) The lesion is round or oval with a base of clean granular tissue over which a crust may form. (3) It is painless or indolent unless pressing on surrounding tissues. (4) When abraided it bleeds only slightly, if at all, after which there is a free flow of serum containing numerous *T. pallida.* (5) The majority of chancres are surrounded by a red non-inflammatory areola. (6) The base and edges of the ulcer become firmly indurated and almost button-hard. This is typical of the 'Hunterian chancre'.

Sites. Chancres have been found on all parts of the body sufrace and within all the orifices, from the top of the head to the tips of the toes, but over 95 per cent occur on the genitalia. In men the commonest sites are the coronal salcus, inner surface of the prepuce, the glans and shaft of the penis. The oedema associated with any subpreputial chancre is sufficient to cause a phimosis, while an intra-meatal sore may cause a serous urethral discharge. In women the majority of genital chancres occur on the vulva, the labia majora or minora, the fourchette and the clitoris, and the cervix. Labial lesions often cause considerable unilateral oedema. Anal chancres are more common than rectal and may appear as indurated fissures rather than as ulcers. They are very rare in women.

In both sexes the commonest sites for extragenital chancres are the lips, where they are often large (up to 2·5 cm in diameter); the tongue; the tonsil, sometimes painful; the fingers, also painful if subungual.

Regional adenopathy

The regional lymph glands usually become enlarged within a week of the appearance of the chancre. They are indolent, discrete, rubbery, globoid and are not adherent to the skin or deeper tissues. They only cause discomfort by their size; in the groin, for example, when walking. The adenopathy associated with chancres of the genitalia and midline structures, while initially unilateral usually becomes bilateral after about a week.

Diagnosis of primary syphilis

The diagnosis of primary syphilis is a laboratory procedure entailing the identification of *T. pallidum* in the serum of chancres or from exudate obtained by gland puncture (See chapter 2). If the results of the initial tests are negative they must be repeated daily for at least 3 days, whithholding all antibiotics and using saline to clean the lesion. The local application of a corticosteroid ointment (0·1 per cent triamcinolone or beta-methasone, or 1·0 per cent hydrocortisone), which encourages the multiplication of treponemes, may be of help in those cases where local antiseptics or antibiotics have been used beforehand. If a microscope with dark ground illumination is not readily available, serum can be transported to a laboratory or special clinic in a capillary tube. Place one end of the tube in the serum and allow 2 to 3 cm to flow in, tap the tube to get the serum into the middle and seal both ends with either candle grease or by heat from a flame. Dark ground microscopy is used to identify *T. pallidum* which, in stained smears fixed by heat, are too thin and mis-shapen to be recognized. With dark ground illumination light is reflected off the edges of the organisms making them appear wider. Thus their morphology, refractile characteristics and movements are more easily visible. *Treponema pallidum* must be distinguished from other treponemes; in the genitalia from *B. refringens, B. gracilis* and *B. balanitidis,* all of which are coarser and more actively motile; in the mouth from *T. macrodentium,* also coarser, and *T. microdentium* which closely resembles *T. pallidum* morphologically but which lacks its rotating and angular movements. Clotted blood should be sent in a dry sterile tube for serological investigations. If exposure to infection has been within a month the laboratory should be asked to carry out the FTA-ABS test, as well as a quantitative VDRL test which will act as a baseline with which to compare subsequent tests carried out after treatment.

Differential diagnosis

The only safe rule is to regard any genital sore or ulcer as syphilitic until proven otherwise, especially if there is a history of exposure to infection. Genital chancres must be differentiated from:

1. *Chancroid.* This ulcerative condition is now rare in temperate climates but remains common in the tropics. The ulcers are painful, multiple and not indurated. They are destructive and bleed easily. The inguinal glands become tender, enlarged and matted, then suppurate (bubo). Dark ground (D.G.) examination is negative, the Ito-Reenstierna skin test is positive, but, of greatest importance, the ulcers heal with sulphonamides.

2. *Herpes genitalis.* Crops of small itchy vesicles develop into superficial ulcers, often with tender inguinal adenitis. The condition is relapsing. D.G. examination is negative and herpes virus can be cultured from scrapings.

3. *Behçet's disease.* Multiple ulcers of the vulva or the scrotum are associated with ulcers in the mouth, lesions in the eyes and fever. D.G. examination and serological tests are negative.

4. *Scabies.* Multiple genital lesions, nodular on the shaft of the penis, may be ulcerated by scratching. Burrows may be seen elsewhere on the body, and a history of nocturnal itching obtained.

5. *Erosive balanitis.* The multiple irregular and tender erosions or ulcers on an inflammatory base are not indurated, although all ulcers in the coronal sulcus appear firm. It is usually found in uncircumcised men and is associated with a purulent subpreputial discharge and a history of some form of trauma. D.G. examination and serological tests are negative.

6. *Other lesions of syphilis.* Eroded papules of secondary syphilis are usually associated with lesions elsewhere and a generalized adenopathy. D.G. examination and blood tests are positive. A punched out gummatous ulcer is deeper than a chancre and without regional adenopathy. D.G. examination is negative and the blood tests positive.

7. *Epithelioma.* This may appear as a chronic ulcer or wart, but bleeds easily, and is found in older, uncircumcised men. It is usually indurated, with a rolled, everted edge and is bound down to the deeper tissues. Metastases in lymph glands are stoney hard. The diagnosis is made by biopsy.

8. *Tuberculous ulceration.* These painful and necrotic ulcerations are very rare. They are usually associated with renal tuberculosis. The diagnosis is made by biopsy.

9. *Lymphogranuloma venereum.* The primary lesion of this tropical sexually transmitted disease is a vesicle or erosion which heals quickly. The associated inguinal adenitis and periadenitis

cause a bubo to form. Inclusion bodies can be identified or *Chlamydia* cultured from the pus. The specific complement fixation test gives a positive result.

10. *Granuloma inguinale.* This is also a tropical sexually transmitted disease. The initial lesion is a painless ulcer which spreads to form a red granulating mass. Donovan bodies are found. in biopsy specimens.

Not every genital lesion is syphilitic, just because the patient has serological evidence of syphilis. Patients with latent syphilis may suffer concurrently from any of the other diseases mentioned. The diagnosis of primary syphilis must be a positive one, by identifying *T. pallidum.*

Extragenital chancres have to be differentiated from a variety of conditions depending on the site of the lesion. Those of the lips and tongue from herpes labialis, aphthous ulcers, Behçet's disease, tuberculosis, epithelioma and trauma, apart from a mucous patch of secondary syphilis or a gumma. A tonsillar chancre may be mistaken for acute tonsillitis, Vincent's angina, infectious mononucleosis, agranulocytosis, lymphosarcoma or a gumma. A primary sore on the nipple may resemble Paget's disease or carcinoma, and on the finger must be distinguished from a simple paronychia, an anthrax pustule, an epithelioma or a sarcoma. On the eyelid an early chancre may be mistaken for a stye. A primary sore at the anus may stimulate a fissure, a thrombosed haemorrhoid or Bowen's disease.

Extragenital chancres are more likely to be missed than those on the genitalia, because the possibility of syphilis is not usually considered by the physician or surgeon concerned. It would be wise routinely to eliminate the possibility of syphilis whenever any of the above conditions are thought to be the most probable diagnosis on clinical grounds alone.

SECONDARY SYPHILIS

The manifestations of the generalized dissemination of *T. pallidum* may occur within a few days of the appearance of the chancre or be delayed for several months. They usually appear about 2 months after infection. During the secondary stage, muco-cutaneous lesions are present in over 80 per cent of cases, enlargement of the lymph glands in over 50 per cent, while less than 10 per cent have lesions of the meninges, bones or joints, eyes, liver and kidneys. The serological tests for syphilis are always positive.

Constitutional symptoms

These are usually mild and affect about 50 per cent of women and 25 per cent of men. They either precede or accompany the onset of the rash, and consist of headaches, especially nocturnal; anorexia, nausea or vomiting, and constipation; muscle or joint pains and aching of the long bones. There may be a low-grade pyrexia. Anaemia and menstrual irregularities are common in women. Persistent occipital headaches with neck stiffness indicate a basal meningitis, jaundice a hepatitis, and while transient albuminuria is common, acute nephritis is rare.

Characteristics of skin lesions

1. *Distribution.* The rash is symmetrical and affects especially the flexor surfaces. In the early stages it is diffuse but later becomes localized with loss of symmetry. The macular or roseolar rash affects the trunk and the limbs but not the face, the palms of the hands or the soles of the feet, all of which are affected by the papular rash.

2. *Colour.* The colour of rashes varies with complexion of the skin. Macules are pink or dusky rose in the centre, fading to the periphery, but are rarely visible in Negroes. Early papules are pink but mature to become 'raw ham', coppery red or 'café au lait.'

3. *Configuration.* The individual lesions are round and initially discrete but become confluent, especially during the florid stage. When the rash is fading the lesions become discrete and then the papules tend to be arranged in circles, or segments of circles.

4. *Induration.* All papules are indurated and feel firm to the extent of each lesion. Those on the palms and soles may even feel shotty.

5. *Symptoms.* Most of the muco-cutaneous lesions are indolent and asymptomatic, but moist papules and condylomata lata at the muco-cutaneous junctions, especially peri-anally, may cause severe itching and burning.

6. *Pleomorphism.* Apart from the early macular stage the rash of secondary syphilis appears in crops, so that papules in various stages of maturity can be found alongside fresh macules in the same area of skin. This is called pleomorphism or polymorphism, and is almost pathognomonic of syphilis.

7. *Pigmentary changes.* While the vast majority of macules and papules heal without leaving a scar, some papules leave pigmented areas which gradually fade. Residual areas of depigmentation,

with surrounding hyperpigmentation, may be found on the skin of the neck (leucoderma colli). These stigma follow the macular syphilide, usually in brunettes.

8. *Adenopathy*. The enlargement of lymph glands is generalized and symmetrical, affecting in particular the posterior cervical, suboccipital, epitrochlear and posterior popliteal as well as the inguinal groups. As in primary syphilis the glands are painless, discrete, rubbery, globoid and non-adherent to surrounding tissues.

Types of skin rashes

Macular or roseolar syphilide. This is usually the initial rash in secondary syphilis. The rose pink colour is best seen in those patients with a pale complexion and is not visible in the Negro. Macules, which are not palpable, disappear under pressure and are round and discrete. They tend to be distributed in the line of the body folds on the trunk and on the flexor surfaces of the limbs. They are best seen in daylight and when the skin is warm, after a hot bath. The eruption may be evanescent or, if it persists, some lesions can become papular giving rise to a mixed maculopapular phase.

Papular syphilides. Papular syphilides develop either from macules or arise as papules. They occur on all the body surfaces and invariably are indurated. The smaller early papules tend to have a diffuse distribution, while the later, larger ones are more localized and arranged in arcs or circles. The colour varies from 'raw ham' to café au lait. Initially the surface is smooth but scales will form if the underlying endarteritis is severe, *squamous syphilide*. With increasing vascular damage pustules may form, *pustular syphilide*, which with central ulceration will become an *impetiginous, ecthymatous* or *rupial syphilide*. In some cases papules spread peripherally, the centre healing, forming an *annular syphilide*. *Eroded papules* develop in warm moist areas, on the scrotum, in the vulva, peri-anally, under pendulous breasts, between rolls of fat and between the toes. With added abrasion and lack of hygiene these eroded papules become confluent, hypertrophic, flattened and 'warty'. These are *condylomata lata*. Initially they are a dull red or pink colour, but with necrosis the surface becomes grey. When this sloughs off it leaves a raw red surface oozing serum heavily laden with treponemes, the most highly contagious lesions of syphilis.

The hair and nails

All skin appendages can be affected during the secondary stage of syphilis. There can be either a generalized thinning of the hair up to complete depilation or an irregular and patchy loss of hair mainly on the back and sides of the head, giving a moth-eaten appearance, *specific alopecia.*

The nails may become brittle and pitted or exfoliated, partially or completely. Papular or pustular lesions of the nail-bed cause crumbling of the nail or a paronychia.

Mucous membrane lesions

Mucous patches. Mucous patches are the equivalent of skin papules on mucous membranes. The surface is eroded by moisture and the lesions are highly contagious. Mucous patches are circular, their flat tops grey-white in colour, with a dull red areola. These non-indurated patches are found within the vulva, sub-prepucially, within the anal canal, on the lips, tonsils, gums, tongue, cheeks and palate. In the mouth they are often associated with a diffuse pharyngitis and laryngitis.

Moist papules. These mainly affect the mucous membranes of the mouth, nose, vulva and anus. They are similar to mucous patches but are more elevated and have an indurated base. Central necrosis is common, causing ulcers with raised edges and red bases. Coalescence of mucous patches or moist papules in a serpiginous formation on the tonsils and surrounding palate gives rise to 'snail track' ulcers.

Diagnosis of secondary syphilis

A cutaneous and/or mucosal eruption should be suspected clinically of being syphilitic when, in the absence of toxaemia, it has the characteristics already mentioned, is associated with a generalized lymphadenopathy and either a chancre or the scar of one. The diagnosis is confirmed by isolating *T. pallidum* from the lesions and the positive results of the STS, the quantitative one at a high titre.

Differential diagnosis

Syphilis can, and does, mimic every form of skin disease, the names of which are often used to describe various syphilitic eruptions: i.e. morbilliform, psoriasiform and framboesiform syphilides.

Macular syphilides. These must be differentiated from measles, rubella, scarlet fever, infectious mononucleosis, erythema multiforme, pityriasis rosea, seborrhoeic dermatitis, drug eruptions and the rose spots of typhoid fever, or flea bites.

Papular syphilides. Smooth papules may simulate chronic urticaria, infectious mononucleosis, urticaria pigmentosa, lichen planus, erythema multiforme, pityriasis rosea and leprosy. *Squamous papules* must be distinguished from psoriasis, seborrhoeic dermatitis and scabies. *Pustular* lesions may be mistaken for smallpox, pustular acne, impetigo, ecthyma, molluscum contagiosum, pyoderma and eruptions due to bromides and iodides. *Annular* lesions can be confused with fungal infections, erythema multiforme, granuloma annulare, lichen planus and impetigo. *Follicular papules* are similar to the lesions of pityriasis rubra pilaris, lichen spinulosis or scrofulosorum on the body, and alopecia areata and ringworm on the scalp. *Condylomata lata* can be misdiagnosed as haemorrhoids, genital warts (*C. acuminata*) and pemphigus vegetans.

The mucosal lesions, *moist papules* and *mucous patches,* have to be differentiated on the genitalia from herpes genitalis, lichen planus, psoriasis, erythroplasia of Queyrat, and in the female from the acute vulval ulcers of Behçet's disease; in the mouth and on the tongue from aphthous ulcers, erythema multiforme, Stevens Johnson syndrome, Behçet's disease, pemphigus, lichen planus, geographical tongue, tuberculous fissures and erosions, herpes simplex, thrush, and drug eruptions due to sulphonamides; on the tonsils and throat from acute tonsillitis, Vincent's angina, infectious mononucleosis and agranulocytosis.

Early latent syphilis

In the absence of any clinical evidence of early syphilis and with normal cerebrospinal fluid findings, early latent syphilis is diagnosed on the basis of confirmed positive results of the specific serological tests for syphilis. It can only be made when there is firm historical evidence that the infection is of less than 2 years duration, such as in the contacts of those suffering from contagious syphilis.

Relapse

With modern therapy relapse is rare, but can occur if treatment is started late and is inadequate. It usually develops within 2 years of treatment, and most commonly at about 6 months. Evidence of treatment failure is always available serologically if searched for. Clinical relapse usually takes the form of secondary lesions, more rarely of a sore at the site of the original chancre. Other indications are the infection of sexual contacts or the birth of a child with congenital syphilis to an apparently cured mother. Non-contagious relapse includes neuro-recurrence, with the appearance of changes in the cerebrospinal fluid not originally present, or clinical evidence of lesions in the eyes, bones, viscera and central nervous system. Clinical relapse is preceeded by serological relapse. Unless a quantitative test is used this will be missed if the various tests did not revert to negative initially. With a quantitative test an initial fall in titre, followed by a persistent and progressive rise indicates serological relapse.

THE MANAGEMENT OF CONTAGIOUS SYPHILIS

Once the diagnosis has been made, and before treatment is discussed, the patient should be interviewed (see chapter 3) about all possible sexual contacts within the past 3 months in the case of primary syphilis, and up to a year for secondary syphilis or 2 years for early latent syphilis. Enquiry should also be made about anyone with whom the patient has been in close bodily contact over a period of time, i.e. sharing the same bed.

It must be impressed on patients that they are contagious and should not have sexual intercourse, marital or otherwise, for one month at least after completing treatment, and then only providing they attend regularly for surveillance. In practice few patients, if any, abstain from intercourse for the 12 months usually advised.

Treatment

Penicillin is the drug of choice, but before it is given or prescribed the patient should be questioned about previous penicillin therapy and any possible reactions, skin rashes, anaphylactoid or of the delayed serum sickness type. If there has been a previous reaction then penicillin is prohibited.

Inquiry should also be made about any personal or familial history of allergic diseases such as hay fever, asthma or urticaria, in which case antibiotics should be used with great care, the patient being best treated in hospital.

Penicillin. The aim is to maintain a blood level of at least

0·03 μg/ml for 15 to 20 days. Oral penicillin is not recommended for two reasons: absorption from the gastro-intestinal tract is uncertain, and reliance has to be placed on the patient taking the stated number of tablets regularly at given intervals. In practice only a few patients carry out their instructions.

Injections of penicillin, or of any other drugs that are released into the blood stream from a depot, should only be given into the upper and outer quadrant of the buttocks, using each side alternately. To ensure that the injection will be given into muscle, and not intravenously, plunge the needle alone, like a dart, into the muscle. Wait to see that blood does not appear from the needle before connecting the syringe to the needle. The injection should be made slowly, the patient either standing up or lying prone, then the needle and syringe together are withdrawn rapidly and the puncture site massaged briskly. Deep intra-muscular injections of procaine penicillin are almost painless. Daily injections of 600 mg (1 mega unit) of procaine penicillin for 10 to 15 days are considered curative for early syphilis. The therapeutic blood level will have been attained within the first day and maintained for over a week after completion of the course. A single injection of 2·4 mega units of benzathine penicillin will give an effective blood level for 2 weeks or more. It is painful, even if half the dose is given into each buttock.

Other drugs. When penicillin cannot be given for whatever cause then cephaloridine 2·0 g daily by intramuscular injection for 10 days can be used, although rare cases of cross-sensitivity with penicillin have been reported. Erythromycin, 500 mg (two tablets) orally ever 6 hours for 15 days is also effective, as are the tetracyclines in a dosage of 750 mg (three tablets) orally every 6 hours for 15 days or doxycycline hydrochloride 100 mg (one capsule) every 8 hours for 10 days. Oral treatment tends to cause bowel upsets including pruritus ani, and should be accompanied by a course of vitamin B (Strong Vitamin B Compound Tablets), B.P.C., one tablet thrice daily.

Untoward reactions to treatment

Occasional reactions do occur and are due to either interaction between penicillin and the patient (hypersensitivity reactions), or any treponemicidal drug and *T. pallidum* (Jarisch-Herxheimer reaction). Reactions are most commonly due to the patient alone (vaso-vagal attacks).

Penicillin

Penicillin is not very toxic. Neurotoxicity, with convulsions or even grand mal seizures, can only occur with very high serum levels associated with renal insufficiency and a diminished blood-brain barrier due to disease in the central nervous system. Nevertheless, penicillin has been so widely used over the past 25 years that a number of people are now sensitive to it. Reactions are due to hypersensitivity, either immediate (anaphylactic) or delayed (toxic-complex syndrome) which occur whether penicillin is applied topically or given systemically. It is an all or nothing phenomenon, developing irrespective of the dose of penicillin.

Less than 5 per cent of patients in Great Britain develop these reactions, but in the United States penicillin is one of the main causes of death due to anaphylaxis. Acute anaphylactic reactions, when mild, cause the patient acute anxiety and fear of impending doom. He may become excited and possibly violent. In severe reactions, immediately after the injection, the patient may stop breathing and collapse pulseless. Death can follow immediately. Delayed reactions may occur at any time from a few hours to a month after the injection, either as redness, urticaria and pruritus localized around the injection site (Arthus reaction), or as a generalized maculo-papular eruption, urticaria and widespread erythema simulating erythema multiforme. Arthralgia with effusions into joints, fever and albuminuria may occur as in serum sickness. Occasionally exfoliative dermatitis or polyarteritis nodosa may follow.

Hypersensitivity reactions can only be prevented if susceptible patients avoid all forms of penicillin. Sometimes there is a previous history of skin or even anaphylactoid reaction, but not always. Tests have been developed to discover hypersensitivity, but as yet none is 100 per cent efficient. Using a solution of 10,000 units of penicillin per ml, 0·2 ml can be injected intradermally or a few drops applied to a scratch on one forearm, saline, in equal quantities, being used as a control on the other arm. A positive result is indicated by a red weal developing within 20 minutes at the test site but not at the control. The test is not without danger as it may itself cause an anaphylactic reaction.

An *in vitro* radio-immunological test, which takes between 36 and 48 hours to perform, has been described. The reagents used in this radio-allergosorbent test (RAST) consist of phenoxymethyl-penicilloyloplylysine (V-PPL) chemically coupled to an insoluble polysaccharide, and an immunosorbent, purified I^{125}-labelled antibodies against IgE. Specific antibodies in the patient's serum react with the V-PPL on the solid matrix and, after washing, these V-PPL bound antibodies are detected by their ability to bind the labelled antibodies to IgE. It is claimed to be as sensitive as the skin test and is of no danger to the patient.

Treatment

Acute anaphylaxis. Wherever penicillin is used as a regular treatment the staff should be trained in the technique of artificial respiration and external cardiac massage, and the necessary equipment for emergency treatment be kept close to hand. The equipment consists of a solution of 1:1,000 adrenaline, amino-phylline, hydrocortisone and an antihistamine for intravenous injection together with phials of distilled water, syringes and needles. An airway, suitable for mouth to mouth respiration, and an oxygen supply should also be readily available.

First aid treatment consists of immediate intramuscular injection of 0·6 ml of 1:1,000 adrenaline, which is a cardiac stimulant and vasoconstrictor. If bronchospasm is present inject 250 mg aminophylline in 10 ml sterile distilled water intravenously. Artificial respiration should be applied using an airway to ensure unimpaired air and oxygen flow and external cardiac massage if necessary. If recovery is not immediate then inject 100 to 250 mg of hydrocortisone or an antihistamine intravenously. If necessary arrange admission for the patient into an intensive care unit for further intravenous therapy with hydrocortisone, nor-adrenaline and plasma during the next 24 hours.

Delayed reactions. These reactions usually respond to a course of oral antihistamines, chlorpheniramine maleate 4 mg three or four times daily or promethazine hydrochloride 25 mg thrice daily. More severe cases may require prednisone or prednisolone, 10 mg four times a day, reducing the dosage gradually after the first few days. If the reaction has been caused by long-acting penicillin, such as benzathine penicillin, it can be eliminated from the body by an intramuscular injection of 1 mega unit of penicillinase, which can be repeated in 2 to 3 days if needed. This treatment is not without danger, as penicillinase itself can cause a reaction, and should therefore be reserved for selected cases.

Jarisch-Herxheimer reaction

This is a systemic and local reaction which affects a proportion of patients on starting treatment for syphilis with any effective treponemicidal drug. The earlier the infection the more frequent and severe are the reactions. Over 50 per cent of patients with contagious syphilis develop a reaction between 6 and 12 hours after the initial treatment. It takes the form of fever, headache, alternating rigors and sweating with aching bones, but the reaction subsides within 24 hours. If present, a chancre swells with oedema and further infiltration. A secondary rash may become apparent or, if already present, become more florid.

The Jarisch-Herxheimer reaction is rare in late syphilis, and is usually limited to a slight rise in temperature. In certain circumstances it can have serious effects; acute oedema in a laryngeal gumma may block the airway, oedema in microgummas can cause occlusion of the coronary ostia or the aqueduct of Sylvius, aneurysms may rupture and arteries, especially cerebral arteries, become thrombosed. In patients suffering from general paresis there may be an increase in psychosis or even epileptiform seizures.

Prevention. There is no treatment for a Jarisch-Herxheimer reaction once it has started, save symptomatic; nor is any needed in early syphilis. Reactions can be prevented or modified by giving prednisolone, 5 mg four times a day during the first 2 days of treatment. In late syphilis, where there is no urgency to start penicillin therapy, reactions can be prevented by giving a course of insoluble bismuth, 0·2 to 0·3 g by intramuscular injection at weekly intervals for 4 to 5 weeks before introducing penicillin therapy.

Vaso-vagal attacks

A number of patients, usually men, feel faint when given an intramuscular injection, or even having a blood test taken. They will quickly recover if given smelling salts, (Spt. ammon. aromat.), 0·3 ml in 20 ml of water to drink and by being laid flat with their clothes loosened.

Surveillance

On completion of treatment the patient should be informed of the need for observation over a period of time, to ensure that the cure will be permanent. Attendance for observation should be at monthly intervals for the first 6 months and then at three-monthly intervals for the next 18 months. If the patient is only in transit, or has to move elsewhere a Personal Booklet of the World Health Organization should be completed, giving details of diagnosis, treatment and surveillance to date, so that surveillance can be completed anywhere throughout the world. At each visit the patient should be questioned about general health, examined for evidence of muco-cutaneous relapse, and blood taken for sero-logical examination. One of the serological tests, preferably the VDRL, should be carried out quantitatively. The reagin tests and the RPCFT usually revert to negative between 3 and 6 months after treatment; the FTA-ABS and TPI tests may take much longer. After one year of surveillance the cerebrospinal fluid is examined. If all the clinical and serological examinations remain satisfactory the patient can be dismissed at the end of the second year.

Prophylactic measures and abortive treatment

There are no effective measures that can be taken prophylac-tically, that is before sexual intercourse, to prevent infection with syphilis. The only certain way is to avoid intercourse with anyone who has had sexual intercourse with a third party within 4 years. Measures taken after sexual intercourse to prevent the develop-ment of syphilis are abortive or suppressive, but not prophylactic as they are sometimes called. None of the local measures, solutions, creams or ointments of antiseptics, disinfectants or antibiotics can be relied upon, nor can washing. They may be effective in some cases but certainly not in all, although they may lull patients into a sense of false security and such agents can themselves cause damage.

Abortive antibiotic treatment of those at risk is not to be advised and still entails full surveillance and the tracing of contacts. Treatment without diagnosis is always second rate medical practice. It is far better to observe contacts for 3 months from risk of infection, when they can be given an absolute assurance of freedom from infection, or if syphilis is diagnosed during this period the patient can be given the treatment appropriate to the findings. There is only one exception to the above rule. If a woman in late pregnancy is a known recent contact of a patient with contagious syphilis, treatment should not necessarily await a full diagnosis, because of the grave risk to the foetus of such delay.

FURTHER READING

Idsøe, O., Guthe, T., Willcox, R. R. & De Week, A. L. (1968). Nature and extent of penicillin side-reactions, with particular reference to fatalities from anaphylactic shock. *Bulletin of the World Health Organization*, **38**, 159.

Kampmeier, R. H. (1946). *Essentials of Syphilology*, 2nd edn. Oxford: Blackwell.

King, A. J. (1965). The treatment of syphilis. *Practitioner*, **195**, 589.

King, A. J. & Nicol, C. (1969). *Venereal Diseases*, 2nd edn. London: Baillière, Tindall & Cassell.

McLachlan, A. E. W. (1947). *Handbook of Diagnosis and Treatment of Venereal Diseases*, 3rd edn. Edinburgh: Livingstone.

Stokes, J. H., Beerman, H. & Ingraham, N. R. (1945). *Modern Clinical Syphilology*, 3rd edn. Philadelphia: Saunders.

Wisdom, A. (1973). *A Colour Atlas of Venereology*. London: Wolfe Medical Books.

8. Late Syphilis

After the early contagious stage of syphilis has run its untreated course, the disease enters its late non-contagious phase about 2 years from infection. Those patients in whom the infection has been latent from the outset and those whose contagious lesions have healed do not usually develop clinical evidence of late syphilis for several years, if ever. During the first few years of late syphilis it can only be transmitted by direct blood transfusion or by a pregnant woman to her foetus but later on, not at all.

LATENT SYPHILIS

The diagnosis of latent syphilis is made by the exclusion of other forms of syphilis, and on the sole basis of serological evidence of syphilis. This entails the repeated positive findings of specific serological tests such as the TPHA, FTA or TPI tests. Elimination of latent cardiovascular and neurosyphilis is made by thorough investigation including, in the cardiovascular system, radiological screening of the heart and aorta and electrocardiographic examination of the heart, and in the central nervous system, examination of the cerebrospinal fluid.

Latent syphilis is usually found by routine screening for syphilis, antenatally, on emigration, and on blood donors. Other cases are discovered from hospital patients in general, those attending with other sexually transmitted diseases or by contact tracing procedures. There is usually a slight preponderance of women with latent syphilis, but a proportion of both men and women do notice an improvement in general health after treatment; it appears that syphilis causes an amount of sub-health as well as ill-health. Latent syphilis must be differentiated from latent congenital syphilis, by the social history and the results of contact tracing, and from latent yaws; this may be almost impossible in certain cases.

BENIGN TERTIARY SYPHILIS

The lesions of benign tertiary syphilis develop between 3 and 10 years after infection. There may be a history of syphilis or other sexually transmitted disease in the past from which to date the infection. Skin, mucous membranes and the underlying tissues, bones, joints, ligaments and muscles can be involved, but the lesions are not lethal, hence the term benign. Certain visceral lesions, however, may be fatal.

Pathology

The typical lesion is a gumma. This is a chronic granulomatous condition sometimes localized, but occasionally diffuse. When localized there is a central area of necrosis surrounded by granulation tissue, and beyond that fibrous tissue. Microscopically the granulation tissue consists of perivascular infiltrations of small lymphocytes, plasma cells, epithelial cells and giant cells. The medial layers of blood vessels degenerate, the intima swells due to the endarteritis and tissues distal to the block become necrosed. Diffuse granulation in the tongue and testes is followed by diffuse fibrosis. Unlike early syphilis the lesions are asymmetrical, either solitary or in clumps, and heal with a scar. In some cases there is a central healing with continued peripheral spread.

Benign tertiary syphilis is found more frequently in women than in men. It is found in association with other forms of late syphilis, with neurosyphilis in 12 per cent and with cardiovascular syphilis in 5 per cent.

Muco-cutaneous lesions

Skin lesions

Cutaneous gummas. These can be either nodular, ulcerative or squamous. The nodular lesions may follow on from the late lesions of secondary syphilis. They tend to be found in clumps or groups, forming arcs or full circles. They are chronic and indolent. Some spread peripherally, leaving a central scar which is atrophic, like 'tissue paper'. Ulcerative lesions develop when there is more marked endarteritis, and the ulcerative edge can become crusted. The most severe endarteritis is associated with squamous lesions, sometimes psoriasiform. On the palms and soles squamous lesions have a waxy and scaling surface.

Subcutaneous gummas. These are round and painless sub-cutaneous swellings, which may be single or multiple. As they increase in size the skin becomes dull red and then breaks down. A punched-out ulcer forms with vertical walls and a wash-leather or dull red granulomatous base. The outline is irregular and the surrounding skin dull red. There is no adenopathy. The ulcers are very slow to heal and leave a 'tissue paper' scar. The common sites are the upper leg, upper trunk, face and scalp.

Mucosal lesions

Gummatous lesions. Localized gummatous lesions are initially submucous and may involve deeper tissues as well as the mucous membrane. Common sites are the palate, pharynx, larynx and nasal septum. At first a painless rounded swelling, the gumma becomes adherent to the mucous membrane which becomes dull red, breaks down with a characteristic wash-leather slough in the base of the ulcer. Palatal gummas usually perforate the hard palate, those of the nasal mucous membrane the septum, while those of the soft palate may destroy the uvula. Ulcerated laryngeal gummas may heal with scarring sufficient to cause laryngeal stenosis, leaving a hoarse and weak voice. All these lesions cause very little discomfort over their chronic course.

Diffuse lesions. These most commonly affect the tongue and more rarely the lips and buccal mucosa. Perivascular interstitial infiltration causes chronic interstitial glossitis. Initially the tongue becomes red, swollen and glazed, and later smooth, glistening and dull red with the loss of the small papillae. Contraction of scars leads either to superficial furrows or deep fissures. For a time the patient may complain of pain associated with hot drinks, spices, vinegar or condiments. Eventually the impaired blood supply leads to patchy necrosis, the adherent epithelium appearing as white areas—leucoplakia. This usually forms on the dorsum of the tongue in syphilis and at the periphery when due to dental irritation. Leucoplakia is a pre-cancerous condition and patients with syphilitic glossitis should be kept under careful observation for many years.

Diagnosis

The diagnosis is made on the clinical appearances, indolent lesions usually ulcerated, together with serological evidence of syphilis. The FTA-ABS and TPHA tests are always positive, the

VDRL and CWR usually so, but the RPCFT may be negative. In addition there may be evidence of syphilis in other systems.

Differential diagnosis. The muco-cutaneous lesions must be differentiated from psoriasis, seborrhoeic dermatitis, bromide and iodide eruptions, and dermatophytosis; other chronic granulomas, tuberculosis, sporotrichosis, blastomycosis and leprosy; Hodgkin's disease, the reticuloses and epitheliomas of the skin. On the face they must be distinguished from lupus vulgaris, rodent ulcer, epithelioma, rhinophyma and leprosy; on the palms from chronic eczema, fungus infections, psoriasis, papulo-necrotic tuberculide and granuloma annulare; on the legs from varicose ulcers, erythema induratum and sporotrichosis.

Lesions of the locomotor system

Bones. Benign tertiary syphilis usually causes an osteoplastic periostitis and, more rarely, an osteoclastic osteitis. The periostitis affects long bones forming irregular swellings, such as the 'sabre tibia'. The cortex is invaded and replaced with sclerotic tissue. Syphilitic osteitis causes destructive lesions in the flat bones, the skull may appear 'worm eaten' radiologically, severe deformity of the palate may cause regurgitation, necrosis of the nasal septum can have the symptoms of oxaena and a supra-clavicular sinus may develop from a gumma at the sternal end of the clavical, which on the left side simulates a broken-down metastatic lymph gland, secondary to carcinoma of the stomach.

Diagnosis

Fifty per cent of bone gummas are associated with nocturnal pain, which is deep and boring in character. When the bones are subcutaneous there will be some swelling and probably tenderness. Gummas of the palate and nasal septum can be diagnosed clinically, but others have radiological appearances that are suggestive. Only on rare occasions do they spread to the subcutaneous tissues and the skin forming ulcers which lead down to necrotic bone: so-called 'syphilitic osteomyelitis'. The serological tests for syphilis are positive as in other types of benign tertiary syphilis.

Differential diagnosis. Syphilitic bone lesions must be differentiated from primary and secondary carcinoma, osteogenic sarcoma, myeloma, Paget's disease, tuberculosis, eosinophilic granuloma, chronic pyogenic osteomyelitis, Ewing's tumor, yaws, leprosy and scurvy.

Primary gummas of muscles, joint, tendon sheaths and bursae are rare but they may be involved from gummas of subcutaneous tissues or bone and if neglected, subsequent scarring may cause contractures. The knee joint, which is subjected to the greatest stress, may be affected by a soft, rubbery, non-inflammatory swelling following the outline of the joint. Hard fibrous juxta-articular nodes may be found in the subcutaneous tissues or on tendon sheaths near joints in late syphilis, and disappear with treatment. The diagnosis of these conditions is made on the basis of the clinical findings and the serological tests for syphilis.

Visceral lesions

All the visceral lesions are considered rare nowadays, but it is probable that they are missed on occasion. Certainly those patients who feel better after being treated for latent syphilis have had lesions too insignificant clinically to be found by routine investigations.

Eyes

While iridocyclitis and chorioretinitis do occur in late secondary syphilis and relapse, they are also found in late syphilis.

Iritis. The symptoms and signs are not specific for syphilis. The patient complains of photophobia, pain and dimness of visions. Examination shows that there is a pink or violet circumcorneal injection, and oedematous iris and a contracted pupil. Later adhesions of the iris can cause a fixed and irregularly contracted pupil.

Chorioretinitis. This is a gummatous infiltration of the choroid which presents as an insidious but progressive loss of vision. In the active phase areas of yellow or grey-white exudate are seen in the retina, which may be cloudy and oedematous. Vitreous opacities may also be present. When scarring occurs blotches of black pigment are seen surrounding white patches, the sclera as seen through the atrophied retina and choroid. Vitreous opacities often mask some of the lesions, which are usually peripheral. The diagnosis is made by the serological results and possibly syphilitic lesions elsewhere. Syphilis must be differentiated from tuberculosis, Reiter's disease, rheumatic infection and focal infection.

Stomach

Gummatous lesions can occur in the stomach but are extremely rare elsewhere in the gastro-intestinal tract. An ulcerating gumma may be associated with hypoacidity and can be symptomatic or not; they are less common in patients with syphilis than are peptic ulcers or carcinoma. Even more rarely a diffuse gummatous infiltration may cause a 'leather bottle' stomach (linitis plastica). The diagnosis of gumma may be made when clinical or radiological improvement follows antisyphilitic therapy.

Liver

The liver is a relatively common site for visceral gummas which are usually multiple and initially cause a hepatomegaly, but during the healing stage sheets and cords of fibrous tissue cause contractions, with the formation of large irregular lobes. This is known as 'hepar lobatum'. Amyloid disease may follow chronic hepatic syphilis. Many liver gummas are asymptomatic but pressure on the bile ducts, gall-bladder or blood vessels, or involvement of the liver parenchyma or capsule can give symptoms. Jaundice, loss of weight, pain and tenderness in the right hypochondrium may occur and be associated with an intermittent fever. Portal hypertension with ascites, anorexia, vomiting and haematemesis from oesophageal varices is very rare. Examination shows a nodular liver, enlarged early and contracted later. The spleen may be enlarged. There is a microcytic anaemia. The liver function tests indicate parenchymatous damage. The diagnosis is sometimes made at laparotomy or by liver biopsy when the patient is being investigated for an obscure liver disease. The serological tests are positive. Syphilis of the liver must be distinguished from secondary carcinoma, hepatoma and carcinoma of the gall-bladder.

Lung

Syphilis rarely affects the lungs and bronchi. Solitary or multiple gummas may simulate tuberculosis or metastases. The symptoms are usually mild with some cough and possibly a little loss of weight, but the scarring may cause a localized bronchiectasis. Usually gummas are diagnosed when a chest X-ray has been taken for other causes. Some patients are subjected to lobectomies, although the diagnosis might have been made on the results of serological findings, and the lesions do respond to treatment.

Genito-urinary tracts

Late syphilis rarely affects the urinary tract, or the genital tract of women. A gumma is occasionally found in the testes, usually as a diffuse interstitial fibrosis, causing a painless smooth swelling with loss of testicular sensation. Occasionally, a localized gumma may involve the subcutaneous tissues and perforate the scrotal skin. The diagnosis of testicular syphilis is by the clinical findings, the serological results and possibly the presence of syphilitic lesions elsewhere. Biopsy will help in the differentiation from neoplasm and tuberculous epididymitis. Mumps and epididymitis are usually acutely painful.

Paroxysmal cold haemoglobinuria

Syphilis is a rare cause of this haemolytic anaemia. Dark brown urine and transient jaundice, associated with headaches, pains, malaise and fever develop when, after exposure to cold, the patient becomes warm again. Red blood cells are broken down by a haemolysin occasionally present in the blood of patients with the benign tertiary syphilis. The haemolysin is activated by cold and acts as an amboceptor, uniting with the red blood cells. When the patient returns to a warm atmosphere the normal complement present in plasma causes the haemolysis. Serological tests for syphilis are positive as is the Donath-Landsteiner reaction, which demonstrates the presence of a haemolysin in the serum; specific serological findings helping to differentiate this from other causes of haemoglobinuria.

The diagnosis of the visceral lesions of late syphilis are usually made when serological tests for syphilis are included in the battery of tests being carried out to find the aetiology of the various symptoms and signs.

CARDIOVASCULAR SYPHILIS

Syphilis is essentially a disease of blood vessels, and of the capillaries and arterioles principally in the contagious and late benign stages. When arteries are affected all the coats are involved, a panarteritis. This condition is rarely diagnosed save in the cerebral and spinal arteries, which will be considered under neurosyphilis. Syphilitic phlebitis is very rare, seen sometimes in late syphilis as a localized and nodular, or diffuse, thickening of the veins. Periphlebitis is occasionally associated with gummatous ulcers of the legs. Syphilis of the heart itself is also rare, but gummas do occasionally affect the myocardium. The most important and commonly diagnosed lesions in the cardiovascular system are those of the aorta and aortic valves, and these are the lesions inferred when discussing cardiovascular syphilis. The signs of cardiovascular syphilis usually take at least 10, and up to 40 years to develop, although the majority of cases are diagnosed within 20 years. One third of the patients also have neurosyphilis and about 7 per cent have benign tertiary lesions. Cardiovascular syphilis is four times more common in men than in women and affects especially Negroes and heavy manual workers.

Pathology

T. pallidum invades the aorta during the first 2 years of the disease by the vasa vasorum. An inflammatory reaction with the perivascular infiltration of small lymphocytes and plasma cells, invades all the coats. Aortitis is most marked in the ascending aorta and the arch which possess a particularly rich lymph supply. In time the adventitia becomes scarred and thickened, but the most serious damage is done in the media where patchy destruction of the elastic and connective tissues leads to fibrosis. This weakens the aortic wall and allows irregular dilatations to develop, up to aneurysmal proportions. The intima is involved and reacts with a compensatory irregular fibrous thickening, giving it a 'tree bark' appearance. Some parts become athero-matous and even ulcerated. Later, calcification supervenes, usually in plaques, but can become so widespread that the aorta is as hard as a drainpipe, but of irregular diameter. The intimal damage spreads down and may affect the coronary ostia, especially if the coronary arteries arise high up in the sinus of Valsalva. Further extension affects the aortic ring causing widening and sagging of the commisures, with separation of the valve cusps. The cusps may be involved, with thickening and rolling-up of their edges, or they may fuse into the aortic wall at the angle of their attachment. There are therefore three causes for aortic valvular incompetence and the diastolic regurgitation of blood into the left ventricle, which has to dilate, and accounts for the low diastolic blood pressure. Compensatory left ventricular hypertrophy develops to the extent allowed by any coronary ostial stenosis, in an effort to propel the increasing amount of blood into the aorta during systole, with a consequent increase in the systolic blood pressure. Left ventricular failure will supervene when the myocardium cannot maintain the blood flow because of coronary insufficiency causing ischaemia, an overwhelming aortic regurgitation, or both.

Uncomplicated aortitis

Uncomplicated aortitis is usually asymptomatic. Rarely a patient will complain of a localized substernal ache. An enhanced aortic second sound like a tambour, or a systolic murmur, in the absence of hypertension or atherosclerosis, in a patient with syphilis indicate aortitis. It can only be diagnosed with certainty by radiological screening. An ordinary X-ray film of the chest may well miss it. Screening shows the irregularities of outline and patches of calcification. Uncomplicated aortitis is usually diagnosed when routine screening of the heart and aorta is carried out on patients thought to be suffering from latent syphilis.

Coronary ostial stenosis

The effects of narrowing of the coronary ostia may be inapparent when there is uncomplicated aortitis, but with the development of aortic incompetence angina pectoris may ensue. This is probably due to the low diastolic aortic blood pressure and irregularities in the blood flow. The patient complains of angina on effort, with emotion or at rest, especially at night. It does not always respond to trinitrin. Complete occlusion is rare, but can cause sudden death. An electrocardiogram may show depression of the $S-T$ segment and inversion of the T-waves over the left ventricle, possibly only detectable when the electrocardiogram is done after exercise.

Aortic incompetence

In the absence of angina and ventricular failure aortic incompetence may remain asymptomatic for many years. Some patients do complain of headache, with a pounding in the ears, but the commonest presenting symptom is dyspnoea. This may be on effort, or paroxysmal and nocturnal. Some patients find that they have to sleep propped up, otherwise they awake breathless and suffocating. This is due to pulmonary oedema, fluid from the legs moving up to the chest when lying in the horizontal position. The first cardinal sign of aortic incompetence is the presence of a Corrigan or water hammer pulse. This is due to the alternating high systolic and low diastolic blood pressures not being damped down in the aorta which is rigid rather than elastic. The Corrigan pulse is best felt by using the palm of the hand, rather than the fingers, against the radial pulse, the wrist being held above the level of the heart. The high pulse pressure can also be demonstrated by capillary pulsation, seen in the finger nail beds or by pressing a glass slide on the everted lips. Examination of the heart usually reveals enlargement, with the apex displaced downwards and outwards. The second cardinal sign of aortic incompetence is the presence of an early diastolic murmur, best heard using the diaphragm of the stethoscope, over the aortic area or down in the left sternal border, but also heard at the apex or even in the axilla, to which it may be transmitted. The murmer is high pitched and diminuendo, less significant than the blowing systolic haemic murmur which accompanies it; together they cause a 'to and fro' murmur. The diastolic murmur can be heard more easily when the patient leans forward having exhaled, and should be timed by the pulse, either of the carotid in the neck or the radial at the wrist. Occasionally blood regurgitating into the left ventricle strikes the aortic cusp of the mitral valve, causing a rough, rumbling mid-diastolic murmur, with presystolic accentuation, heard at the apex. This is known as the Austin-Flint murmur. Radiological examination may show enlargement of the left ventricle, unfolding of the aorta and calcification, best seen by screening. The electrocardiogram is sometimes normal, even after exercise, but usually shows left axis deviation due to left ventricular strain and later depression of the $S-T$ segments and inverted T-waves in the chest leads over the left ventricle.

Differential diagnosis

Syphilitic aortic incompetence must be differentiated from other causes of aortic incompetence, Reiter's disease, ankylosing spondylitis, Marfan's syndrome, congenital bicuspid aortic valve, and atherosclerosis with calcification of the aortic valve, all of which lack aortitis. Pulmonary hypertension may cause a diastolic murmur but lacks the peripheral signs, which are present in patent ductus arteriosus but which has a continuous murmur. Rheumatic heart disease usually causes aortic stenosis and there is an associated mitral disease. Bacterial endocarditis usually complicates rheumatic heart disease.

Heart block

A gumma situated in the interventricular septum is a rare cause of incomplete or complete heart block. Heart block in patients with syphilis is more commonly due to intercurrent rheumatic heart disease, atherosclerosis, myocardial infarct or digitalis effect than to a gumma, which does carry a better prognosis.

Aneurysms of the aorta

Aneurysm of the ascending aorta

Syphilitic aneurysms can be either fusiform or saccular. The latter tend to become partially filled with blood clots which become organized, and are sources of emboli. The endothelium lining aneurysms usually becomes ulcerated and calcified. They are always liable to rupture. The commonest site for a syphilitic aneurysm is in the first part of the aorta, where it is known as the 'aneurysm of signs'. If it bulges laterally it will press on the right lung causing dullness on percussion and a loud systolic murmur. An anterior bulge will press on the ribs and sternum, presenting as a pulsating mass when they become eroded. Extension medially will cause pressure on the trachea or pulmonary artery, and this can cause right heart failure. Death may occur due to rupture into the pleura, pericardium, trachea or through the skin.

Aneurysm of the arch of the aorta

Aneurysms of the second part of the aorta are known as 'aneurysms of symptoms'. They usually arise from the convex surface, press on structures in the superior mediastinum and present as a pulsating mass in the suprasternal notch. Pressure on the trachea causes stridor and a brassy cough, on the oesophagus dysphagia, on the left bronchus possible collapse of the lung and tracheal tug. Haemoptysis can be due to tracheal congestion or an aneurysmal leak. Stretching of the left recurrent laryngeal nerve causes paralysis of the left vocal cord, with hoarseness, and of the sympathetic nerves Horner's syndrome, unilateral meiosis, enophthalmos and ptosis. In addition sweating may be impaired on the same side of the face. Paralysis of the diaphragm may occur if the phrenic nerve is involved. Distortion of the vessels arising out of the arch and pressure on them may cause inequality of the pulses in the arms. Compression of the superior vena cava will cause cyanosis, oedema and congestion of the veins of the head, neck and upper chest. Death can occur from rupture into the trachea, pleura, pericardium and mediastinum.

Aneurysm of the descending aorta

Aneurysms of the descending aorta are usually silent. Occasionally there may be a persistent boring pain in the back. Lateral X-rays of the chest may show erosion of the vertebrae with sparing of the intervertebral discs. Syphilitic aneurysms are generally confined to the thorax, they are very rare in the abdomen, and do not tend to rupture.

Diagnosis

In some cases the symptoms and signs are so suggestive that a clinical diagnosis of aneurysm can be made with confidence. Nevertheless radiological confirmation should always be obtained. This is best done by means of screening, during which films can be taken for comparison with others done at a later date. Barium swallow, tomography and angiocardiography may be needed on occasion to differentiate aneurysms from other space-occupying, non-vascular, thoracic lesions which are usually due to malignant disease.

NEUROSYPHILIS

Treponema pallidum can be found in the cerebrospinal fluid from the time that the chancre appears. Between 30 and 40 per cent of patients with secondary syphilis have changes in the cerebrospinal fluid, although few develop acute syphilitic meningitis. The vast majority of these patients are cured with routine treatment, while of those untreated, only about 10 per cent develop late clinical neurosyphilis. This may take many years; in the meantime the neurosyphilis remains latent. During the first 5 to 7 years the disease affects mainly the meninges and blood vessels, so-called non-parenchymatous neurosyphilis, and recovery can be expected after treatment. Later on the brain and spinal cord parenchyma are damaged and treatment is followed by only limited recovery, if any. Neurosyphilis is twice as common in men as in women but is found less frequently in Negroes than in the other races.

Cerebrospinal fluid examination

Examination of the cerebrospinal fluid is mandatory in the diagnosis or elimination of neurosyphilis and should be carried out before treatment in all except contagious cases. Certain tests are obligatory: a cell count, a test for globulin, total protein estimation, serological tests and the colloidal gold test. If necessary individual laboratories should be requested not to waste valuable cerebrospinal fluid on sugar and chloride estimations which are not affected in neurosyphilis. Certain tests can be carried out by the clinician; the cell count is normally three or less lymphocytes per mm^3. The presence of five or more lymphocytes, or one polymorphonuclear leucocyte is considered pathological. The presence of an excess of globulin is also pathological. This can be determined by the Nonne-Apelt method; equal parts of cerebrospinal fluid and a hypersaturated solution of ammonium sulphate are mixed in a tube. Any haze indicates an excess of globulin, which may be present when there is only a slight increase in protein above the accepted upper normal level of 40 mg per 100 ml. Neurosyphilis can be graded according to the severity of the abnormal cerebrospinal fluid findings. This is of prognostic value not only in the management of latent infections but also of the various clinical syndromes.

Table 4 Grading of abnormal cerebrospinal fluid findings in neurosyphilis

	Grade I	Grade II	Grade III
Cells per mm^3	5–25	25–100	7–100+
Globulin	Negative or positive	Positive(+)	Positive(++)
Protein	Normal or increased	Increased(+)	Increased(++)
Reagin tests	Negative	Positive at low titre	Positive at high titre
Colloidal gold test	1110000000 or 0000011000	0024454310 mid-zone curve	5555543100 first zone curve
Reagin tests in the serum	Negative or weakly positive	Weakly positive or positive	Positive at high titre

A Grade III cerebrospinal fluid carries the most severe prognosis, the patient requiring thorough treatment, without which general paresis may develop. It should be remembered that the cerebrospinal fluid findings only reflect active pathological processes, either inflammatory or degenerative, in tissues adjacent to it, and that normal results may be obtained when the condition is 'burnt out', deep seated or of very low activity.

Acute syphilitic meningitis

This may occur during the course of secondary syphilis but is more likely during relapse. Usually it is more of a meningism, with headache and neck stiffness only, but severe cases have pyrexia, convulsions and coma. Vomiting and papilloedema indicate raised intracranial pressure. Ocular palsies, especially of the external rectus which is supplied by the abducent nerve, occur more frequently than deafness. Examination of the cerebrospinal fluid shows a marked pleocytosis, of up to 1000 lymphocytes per mm^3, the presence of globulin and a moderate increase in protein. Often the reagin tests are negative and the colloidal-gold curve normal. Serological tests with blood serum are all positive and those done quantitatively positive at high titre.

Latent neurosyphilis

This is sometimes called asymptomatic neurosyphilis, but it is only diagnosed in the absence of both symptoms and signs. The diagnosis is entirely a laboratory procedure, the severity of the damage being gauged from the grading of the cerebrospinal fluid. Because of the potential danger of latent neurosyphilis with Grade III findings it is sometimes known as 'paresis sine paresis' or 'paresis imminens'. Latent neurosyphilis includes cases of both non-parenchymatous and parenchymatous damage, and may be diagnosed at any time from three to thirty years from infection. It may be found in 15 per cent of those initially diagnosed as latent syphilis, in 13 per cent of those with cardiovascular syphilis, and in 5 per cent of those with benign tertiary syphilis.

Non-parenchymatous neurosyphilis

The non-parenchymatous lesions are sometimes referred to as meningo-vascular neurosyphilis. Both the meninges and blood vessels are affected but usually the symptoms and signs in an individual case are predominantly due to damage of one or the other.

Mainly meningeal

The pia and arachnoid are principally affected with perivascular infiltration of small lymphocytes and plasma cells followed by fibrosis. Inflammation of the ependyma is followed by subependymal gliosis, which may affect the tract carrying the light reflex to the fore brain. The inflammatory process spreads from the meninges into the cortex of the brain and the nerve tracts of the spinal cord, especially the motor tracts causing a meningomyelitis. The meningitis or the subsequent scars may compress the infranuclear tracts of the cranial and spinal nerves producing lower motor-neurone lesions.

Symptoms and signs. When the cortex is involved the symptoms are of mild headache, often nocturnal, slight dizziness, insomnia, general lassitude and poor concentration, but may be severe with intense headache, neck stiffness and blurred vision. Mental confusion can be as severe as in general paresis and associated with epileptiform seizures. When the vertex is involved there may be aphasia, papilloedema, monoplegia or hemiplegia. Basal meningitis may cause palsies of the 3rd, 6th, 7th, or 8th cranial nerves. The light reflex may be lost and the pupils contracted, sometimes unequally. Contracted pupils which do not react to light but do to accommodation, or convergence, are almost pathognomonic of neurosyphilis, and were originally described by Argyll Robertson.

Spinal meningitis and myelitis are less common and the clinical onset is insidious. In the cervical region a hypertrophic pachymeningitis, involving the nerve roots and spinal tracts, causes bulbar symptoms, Horner's syndrome and headaches. There is weakness and areflexia of the shoulder girdle and arms, and spastic paraplegia may eventually develop. Amyotrophic lateral sclerosis will cause lower motor-neurone lesions of the shoulder girdle, arms and the small muscles of the hands. Spastic paraplegia is rare. Damage to the pyramidal tracts by a dorsolumbar meningitis causes Erb's spastic paraplegia. The early symptoms are of stiffness of the legs and either frequency of micturition or retention of urine, due to bladder sphincter disturbance. Paraesthesiae may also occur. There is increased tone in the muscles, and the reflexes are enhanced. Ankle clonus and extensor plantar responses are often found. The cerebrospinal fluid findings are usually moderately severe; Grade II or, rarely Grade I. All of the serological tests are positive.

Differential diagnosis. Cerebral meningitis must be differentiated from other causes of meningitis; space-occupying lesions, such as tumours, abscesses and gumma; other causes of raised intracranial pressure; epilepsy and mental disease including general paresis. Spinal meningitis may be confused with multiple sclerosis, tumours, disc lesions or other motor-neurone disease.

Mainly vascular

Endarteritis affects the medium-sized cerebral and spinal arteries with narrowing of the lumen and a liability to thrombosis. The middle and posterior cerebral arteries and their branches are most commonly affected, but the anterior cerebral, cerebellar and basilar arteries can also be affected as well as the spinal arteries, but much more rarely. Partial occlusion is common and recovery from early episodes usual. Initially the symptoms are mild; headaches, dizziness and possibly some clouding of the consciousness, but rarely unconsciousness. Usually the early episodes are only transitory, paresis of a limb or the face with recovery within a day or so, but eventually an attack will leave permanent damage. Such a history in a young, or middle-aged person, without hypertension or atherosclerosis is very suggestive of vascular neurosyphilis. Hemiplegia is the commonest manifestation of cerebral attacks, but mental deterioration, motor aphasia, hemianaesthesia, hemiathetosis, hemianopia and dysphagia may be found according to the site of the arterial occlusion. Sudden flaccid paralysis with loss of sphincter control and later spastic paraplegia can be caused by spinal artery thrombosis. The cerebrospinal fluid findings are mild, either Grade I or normal. The serum reagin tests are usually positive.

Differential diagnosis. Cerebral vascular syphilis must be differentiated from cerebral thrombosis due to atherosclerosis and hypertension. Spinal vascular syphilis from transverse myelitis, tumours and gummas. Vascular syphilis should be distinguished from meningeal syphilis, although a number of patients have signs and symptoms of both.

Parenchymatous neurosyphilis

Syphilis affects the parenchyma of the brain causing general paresis and of the spinal cord producing tabes dorsalis. When there is evidence of both cerebral and spinal damage the condition is called tabo-paresis.

General paresis

General paresis is also known as general paralysis of the insane or dementia paralytica, titles which date from the time when mental hospitals were filled with these helpless and hapless patients. Nowadays paretic patients, who are often demented and occasionally insane, do not become generally paralysed. General paresis is now uncommon in mental hospitals. The clinical onset is usually between 7 and 20 years after infection, the majority of patients being in their thirties and forties. It is more common in Europeans, or Caucasians, than in other races, and in men than women. A proportion of patients also have cardiovascular syphilis.

Pathology. At necropsy the dura mater is found to be thickened and adherent to the skull. The pia is opaque, thickened and adherent to the cortex, and on removal leaves a 'worm eaten' surface. The brain is shrunken and the convolutions wasted, especially those of the frontal and middle lobes, which are firm because of gliosis. The atrophy is mainly of the white matter, the grey matter being reddened from increased vascularity. The ventricles are dilated and the cerebrospinal fluid volume increased to fill them and the larger subrachanoid space. The ependyma is granular and there are glial granulations on the floor of the fourth ventricle. Microscopically there is perivascular infiltration of the arterioles of the meninges and of those entering the brain. There is a reduction in the number of ganglion cells, degeneration of nerve cells and demyelination of fibres in the cortex with gliosis. The storage of an iron-containing substance in the microglia is considered pathognomonic of general paresis. *Treponema pallidum* can be identified in the cortex, using special staining methods, in about 50 per cent of cases coming to necropsy.

Symptoms. The onset of mental symptoms may be so insidious that they are not noticed by the patient, and only by the relatives after a time. They often seek aid when they fear that the patient is about to have a 'nervous breakdown'. Initially the patient loses concentration and some memory; he tires easily and becomes increasingly unstable. While easily annoyed by others he has no insight into his own problem. Headaches and insomnia may be followed by persistent drowsiness. The patient may complain of tiredness or being 'off colour' but rarely more. Personality changes develop, and always for the worse; behaviour deteriorates, judgment becomes increasingly defective, the appearance is unkempt and the habits dirty. The patient may become emotionally labile, having weeping fits without apparent cause and temper tantrums during which he may cause a breach of the peace. On occasion the onset of general paresis can be acute, with sudden epileptiform seizures or convulsions followed by transient hemiparesis and aphasia, but usually the earliest symptoms have the appearance of neurasthenia, later of neurosis and finally of psychosis with dementia. Depression is commonly found in these demented patients, delusions of grandeur are rarely seen nowadays.

Signs. Pupillary changes are the commonest signs in general paresis. About 25 per cent have Argyll-Robertson pupils, but many more have other abnormalities, inequality, irregularity, sluggish reaction to light or fixed and usually contracted pupils. Ophthalmoplegia may be present but optic atrophy is only found in the presence of tabes, in tabo-paresis. Tremors are often one of the early signs, those of the face around the mouth and eyelids, and of the hands, being fine, while that of the tongue is slower and coarser, being known as a 'trombone' tremor. The facial expression is vacuous, lacking emotion, and the skin creases tend to fade. Speech is indistinct and tremulous, a slurred dysarthria, best brought out when the patient has to keep repeating a test phrase such as 'British Constitution' or 'Artillery Brigade'. In addition there may be a nominal aphasia. Routine testing should be done to elicit this and the amount of intellectual impairment by simple arithmetical problems, addition and subtraction, by questions of general knowledge and by the patients' ability to write, at dictation, a sentence or two. In general paresis the handwriting becomes shaky and deteriorates. Words are misspelt and often sentences end meaninglessly. Degeneration of the pyramidal tracts causes exaggerated tendon reflexes in all the limbs, absent or diminished abdominal reflexes and extensor plantar responses. Ultimately, but very rarely, spastic paraplegia may supervene. Incontinence of both urine and faeces may occur relatively early and is due to mental deterioration, not to sphincter disturbances. In cases of tabo-paresis there will be signs of posterior column involvement.

The cerebrospinal fluid findings are almost always Grade III unless antibiotics have been given recently, in which case they may be Grade II. All of the serological tests for syphilis are always positive.

Differential diagnosis. The symptoms of general paresis are neurasthenic initially, then neurotic and finally psychotic. General paresis must be distinguished from the psychoses associated with schizophrenia, manic depressive psychosis, cerebral atherosclerosis, senile dementia and the presenile dementias of Pick and Alzheimer; from encephalitis, miliary tuberculosis and multiple sclerosis; the toxic effects of alcohol, drug addiction and liver failure; subacute combined degeneration of the cord, epilepsy, subdural haematoma, Huntingdon's chorea, heart failure, carcinomatosis and cerebral tumours. Differentiation of any of these from general paresis may be difficult in a patient with latent neurosyphilis, while meningovascular syphilis may only be distinguished by its response to treatment.

Tabes dorsalis

Tabes dorsalis is sometimes known as locomotor ataxis. It is characterized pathologically by degeneration of the posterior columns and roots of the spinal cord, and clinically by numerous symptoms including ataxia, pain and sensory changes, loss of deep reflexes and trophic changes; also by changes in the special senses and the pupils. This disease is twice as common in men as in women, and accounts for about a third of all cases of neurosyphilis. The clinical manifestations rarely occur within 10 years of infection and may take up to 30 or more. Evidence of concomitant general paresis or cardiovascular syphilis will be found in a proportion of patients with tabes dorsalis, which can be divided into stages: pre-ataxic, ataxic, and finally, in a few cases only, paralytic.

Pathology. Macroscopically there is sclerosis in the posterior columns which become flattened, grey and translucent, especially in the dorso-lumbar region, where the arachnoid becomes thickened and opaque. Microscopically there may be a perivascular infiltration of the posterior nerve roots where they pierce the meninges, the pia and arachnoid also being affected. Later, atrophy of the posterior nerve roots with degeneration between the ganglion and the cord will be found. There is an ascending degeneration of the posterior columns with an increase in microglia. The essential lesion is a primary progressive degeneration of the posterior root fibres after entering the cord, the cause of which is probably the inflammatory process of the pia on the dorsum of the cord, which crushes the fibres at the point where a natural constriction normally occurs on entering the cord. It is not now thought that syphilitic toxins attack the fibres which have just lost their neurolemma sheaths on entering the cord. Spinothalamic conduction may be impaired and the autonomic nervous system is also involved. Degenerative changes can occur in any sensory nerve, the most commonly affected being the trigeminal and glosspharangeal nerves. Primary optic atrophy may be caused either by a primary degeneration of the retinal ganglion cells or a gummatous neuropathy of the optic nerve.

Symptoms. The onset may be insidious and over a period of years. Symptoms are numerous and any one of them may be the first to appear, or be noticed by the patient. The most characteristic of the pains associated with tabes dorsalis are called 'lightning' pains. They are intense and stabbing in nature, come in bouts over a period of minutes, hours or days, separated by periods of complete freedom from pain lasting days, weeks or months, and they usually affect the legs. They often seem to enter and leave the limb at right angles to the skin surface. They are not provoked by exercise, but rather by the weather, indigestion and any intercurrent infection. When severe they may be associated with localized skin vasodilatation. The intensity of the pains can vary from only slight discomfort to such utter agony that suicide may be attempted. Some patients complain of formication, the feeling that little things are crawling under the skin, and these can be equally distressing. Girdle pains, the unpleasant sensations of a tight band around the trunk, especially of the upper abdomen, may occur or even trigeminal neuralgia, usually of the mandibular division, with dull spasms lasting a few seconds, in bouts which may last for days or weeks and recur at intervals. 'Rheumatism', with aches or cramps in the muscles rather than pain, may be prolonged in some cases of tabes dorsalis, while in others there are burning sensations on the soles of the feet. Far more patients feel that they are walking on cotton wool, and while anaesthesia may affect the legs, sometimes in a stocking distribution, the trunk and a 'butterfly' area over the nose may also be affected. Hyperaesthesia and paraesthesia in these areas may be noted by other patients.

Bladder disturbances occur when the sacral roots are affected. This may be early in the disease. Loss of bladder sensation leads to over-distention with increased intravesical pressure, at a critical level of which urine is voided automatically and without warning.

With chronic over-distention the critical pressure rises and the amount of residual urine increases. The urine often becomes infected and this may lead to recurrent attacks of pyelonephritis, a common cause of death, especially in women. Chronic stretching of the detrusor muscle causes difficulty in starting micturition and a poor stream. In time the stream becomes intermittent and later retention with overflow may follow. Impotence, or diminished libido and potency, may be another early symptom when the sacral roots are involved. Chronic constipation, due to diminished tone of the colon, is common but faecal incontinence, due to atonic sphincters is rather rare. When present, it is usually due to general paresis.

Painless failing vision may be an early and isolated symptom. Primary optic atrophy may have a gradual onset, affecting one eye in particular, or be bilateral, and cause rapid blindness, even within a month of onset. It depends on whether there is initial constriction of the peripheral fields or a central scotoma. Many patients with syphilitic primary optic atrophy do not develop any other tabetic lesions.

Tabetic, or visceral, crises are paroxysms of pain in various organs due to damage to the automic nervous system. They may be an early manifestation of tabes dorsalis. The most common are gastric crises which begin with epigastric pain, anorexia and vomiting. They may last for up to 2 days, after which the symptoms suddenly stop, but recurrences are frequent. Occasionally there are prodromal symptoms of vague abdominal pains, or the pain, during a crisis, may be in the lower abdomen. Crises also occur in the rectum, with severe rectal pain and tenesmus; in the bladder, with pain in the penis or clitoris; in the kidney, with pain in the loins. Laryngeal crises cause attacks of stridor, both inspiratory and expiratory, cough and severe dyspnoea, sufficient to warrant tracheotomy on occasions.

Tabetic ataxia, with instability and an unsteady gait, is worse when vision cannot help to maintain balance. It is usually a late symptom and is due to loss of postural sense. Ataxia is noted when washing the face or when in the dark. The patient may notice that he has to walk with feet wide apart on a broad base and that the feet have to be raised high to avoid stubbing the toes when walking on uneven surfaces such as cobble stones. Ataxia progresses as the ability to co-ordinate movements deteriorates, so that the patient can neither walk nor stand without the aid of a stick. Later even that becomes impossible, and the patient is then immobilized. Finally, and only in a very few cases, the trunk becomes affected so that the patient cannot even sit upright unaided. This represents the paralytic stage. The upper limbs are only rarely affected to any extent, ataxia being manifest by an increasing clumsiness of the fingers, hands and arms. Complete upper limb paralysis is extremely rare.

The symptoms of trophic lesions usually occur during the ataxic stage. Painless instability and swelling of a joint, a Charcot's neuropathic arthropathy, usually has an insidious onset. The joint, or joints, affected are usually weight bearing. Thickened skin, like a corn, may develop on the sole of a foot at a pressure point, usually under the big toe. A painless trophic ulcer, penetrating deeply and involving the underlying bone, may develop, especially if the patient has attempted to remove the corn. Sudden weakness with a variable amount of local pain and without a history of trauma may be due to a pathological fracture, especially in post-menopausal women.

Signs. Patients with tabes dorsalis are usually thin and often appear to be undernourished. The skin is pale and the muscles flabby. Hypotonia and an unequal ptosis, with a compensatory wrinkling of the forehead on the affected side, give the typical 'tabetic facies'. Pupillary abnormalities are present in almost every case of tabes dorsalis. The pupils may be irregular, unequal or contracted and react normally or sluggishly to light. Argyll-Robertson pupils may be present bilaterally, or one pupil may retain a sluggish reaction to light. Some pupils, having passed through the Argyll-Robertson stage, are contracted and fixed to both light and accommodation or convergence. Primary optic atrophy occurs in about 20 per cent of tabetics. The optic disc is pale and stands out against the red fundus. The margin is sharply defined and there is an absence of small vessels on the disc. Examination of the visual fields usually shows concentric constriction; a central scotoma is rare.

Evidence of posterior column damage will be found mainly in the lower limbs. Hypotonia, or later atony, may be such that the tabetic can perform contortions. Loss of muscle power is usually minimal. Tendon reflexes become diminished and later lost, at the ankles before the knees, but only very rarely in the upper limbs. The plantar responses remain flexor throughout. While the cremasteric reflexes may be lost early, the abdominal reflexes usually remain intact unless there is hypotonia of the abdominal muscles.

Often there is early loss of those modalities of sensation transmitted by the posterior columns. Loss of deep pain is demonstrated by squeezing the Achilles tendon, the testes, and the ulnar nerve trunk at the elbow. Vibration sense may be lost over the sternum as well as the lower limbs. Loss of joint position sense prevents the tabetic from knowing the position of the toes when passively moved up or down, unless he can see them. Changes in skin sensation include diminution or loss of sensation to pin prick or touch, or lack of discrimination between them. There may be analgesia or anaesthesia around the nose, over the sternum, on the inner sides of the forearms, the lateral surfaces of the legs and in the perianal region. Occasionally, sensory loss is over a 'stocking' or 'girdle' area. In some cases there is an appreciable delay in pain conduction, or loss of localization of the pin prick. Hyperaesthesia may be present over the flanks and on the soles of the feet.

Palpation of the abdomen may reveal a grossly distended bladder, pressure upon which shows that there is retention with overflow. Trabeculations can be seen by cystoscopy, at which time the residual urine can be measured and a portion examined bacteriologically for infection. The hypotonia can be measured cystometrically. Impacted faeces may be found on rectal examination and are evidence of constipation due to colonic hypotonia.

Charcot's arthropathy is caused by the neuropathic changes occurring in tabes dorsalis. A joint relies for its stability on the tension of the tendons and muscles inserted around it. A Charcot's joint will develop when stability is lost due to hypotonia if, in addition, there is ataxia, with unco-ordinated movements. Over a period of time this causes repeated trauma, unnoticed because of the lack of joint pain, to the articular cartilage and underlying bones which have a deficient blood supply, because of the tabetic damage to the autonomic nervous system. Initially the cartilage becomes thin and eroded; the underlying bone is destroyed and becomes sclerosed. At the same time peripheral exostoses develop due to the periosteal reaction. Loose bodies are formed because of the avascular necrosis. Ultimately the joint becomes disorganized and has abnormal movements without pain. The weight-bearing joints are most commonly affected, the knee, ankle, foot, spine and hip in that order of frequency. Sometimes more than one joint is affected, but it is rarely bilateral. Examination of a Charcot's joint shows that there is an excess of fluid and a painless coarse crepitus, that can not only be felt, but on occasions heard also. Passive movements may be so abnormal that the joint can be dislocated, this is a flail joint. Radiological examination may show widening of the joint space, thinning of the cartilage, subchondral sclerosis, exostoses with periosteal reaction, foreign bodies, disorganization of the joint and possibly pathological fractures of the adjacent bones. A trophic ulcer under the big toe is called a 'mal perforans'. It is very chronic, indolent and, in time, often penetrates to the bone or joint beneath. Pyogenic infection may cause an osteomyelitis or destruction of the metatarso-phalangeal joint, conditions which are usually diagnosed radiologically.

The cerebrospinal fluid findings are usually Grade II, but in about 30 per cent of patients the conditions will be 'burnt out', and the cerebrospinal fluid findings normal. Half of these patients will also have negative reagin tests in the serum. The overall incidence of negative reagin tests in the blood is about 25 per cent. The FTA-ABS test is almost always positive, the TPI test so in about 80 to 90 per cent of cases.

Differential diagnosis. Tabes dorsalis must be differentiated from other neurological conditions; peripheral neuropathies associated with alcoholism, diabetes mellitus, infectious poly-neuritis, vitamin deficiencies, lead poisoning and diphtheria; subacute combined degeneration of the cord; multiple sclerosis; Friedreich's ataxia; peroneal muscular atrophy; cerebellar degenerations; tumours of the cauda equina. In addition certain manifestations of tabes must be distinguished from other conditions. Gastric crises and root pains of the trunk from abdominal surgical emergencies, e.g. perforated peptic ulcer, acute cholecystitis or appendicitis. Atonic bladder from prostatic hypertrophy or urethral stricture. Charcot's joints from syringo-myelia or osteoarthritis. Mal perforans from diabetic neuropathy. Trigeminal neuralgia and optic atrophy from other causes of these conditions. Argyll-Robertson pupils, absent or diminished knee and ankle jerks may be confused with Adie's syndrome, a benign condition not associated with disease of the central nervous system, and in which usually one pupil is myotonic and larger than normal. With ordinary testing there is no reaction to light, but in the dark there is slow dilatation and in the light slow contraction. The pupil dilates fully with mydriatics and there is no degeneration of the iris. The condition is more common in young women than middle-aged men but a number of people with this pupil reaction do have diminished or absent tendon reflexes in the lower limbs.

Gumma

Benign tertiary lesions of the brain and spinal cord are very rare. Gummas usually develop from the meninges and produce symptoms and signs by pressure upon neighbouring structures. They can occur anywhere. In the brain they may cause an increased intracranial pressure, with headache, nausea and vomiting, convulsions especially temporal, or a progressive diminution of vision. Examination may show papilloedema, but localizing signs will depend on the site of the lesion. An encephalogram may locate a silent gumma. In the spinal cord gradual but increasing pressure on the cord may produce spastic paraplegia with a well-defined level of sensory loss. Trophic ulcers only occur rarely. A gumma blocking the spinal canal can cause Froin's syndrome: below it there is such an excess of protein that the cerebrospinal fluid is thickened. The differential diagnosis is from other space-occupying lesions. It may be difficult to differentiate from a cerebral tumour except by biopsy, unless the cerebrospinal fluid is examined and serum serological tests carried out. The cerebrospinal fluid findings are usually either Grade I or II and the serum serological tests positive.

THE MANAGEMENT OF LATE SYPHILIS

Once the diagnosis of late syphilis has been established arrangements should be made for the examination of the marital partner, and if the patient is a woman, her children also. It is worth while questioning patients to see if they can remember having had lesions of early syphilis in the past, and if so do they know any possible contacts from that time. On occasions untreated, but apparently healthy contacts will be discovered who otherwise would have to await diagnosis until symptoms and signs eventually develop.

Latent syphilis

In the absence of clinical evidence of syphilis, other than the scars of past contagious syphilis, the diagnosis is made by the elimination of latent cardiovascular and neurosyphilis, using the appropriate tests. The serological diagnosis must be made on the basis of the results of specific tests. Unless penicillin is contraindicated, a course of procaine penicillin 600 mg (1 mega unit) daily by deep intramuscular injection for 10 to 15 days should suffice. If penicillin cannot be used, cephaloridine, 2·0 g daily for 10 days, can be given by deep intramuscular injection. Erythromycin, 500 mg (two tablets), or one of the tetracyclines, 750 mg (three tablets), orally every 6 hours for 15 days is also effective, but should only be given under strict supervision.

A number of patients can be expected to feel in better health after treatment, indicating that there have been active lesions not identified during the pre-treatment investigations. Serological surveillance should be at monthly intervals for the first 6 months after treatment and then at three-monthly intervals up to 5 years. Further annual examinations for many years should be advised for those patients in whom the reaction of any of the tests remains doubtful or positive, although the prognosis is excellent.

Benign tertiary syphilis

Having eliminated a concurrent cardiovascular or neurosyphilis, a course of antibiotics similar to that for latent syphilis is effective in the treatment of benign tertiary syphilis. An introductory course of bismuth will prevent the possibility of a Jarisch–Herxheimer reaction (see p. 87) on starting subsequent antibiotic therapy. Time will not have been wasted as there is no urgency in starting treatment for syphilis of many years' duration. Insoluble bismuth is given by deep intramuscular injection, 0·2 to 0·3 g weekly for 4 or 5 weeks, bearing in mind that bismuth is contraindicated in cases of pyorrhoea and kidney disease. Iodides, in the form of a mixture containing potassium iodide, may help in the healing of gummatous lesions, especially of bones. The dose is increased from 0·6 to 2·0 g three times a day.

Once the lesions have healed plastic surgery may be needed, for cosmetic reasons on the face or to remove deep scars interfering with mobility. Perforations of the palate may need repairing or covering with a dental plate. Serological surveillance is as for latent syphilis, and the prognosis is usually very good indeed, but if clinical or serological response is considered inadequate, a further course of treatment may be given. Some prefer to use a long-acting penicillin such as benzathine penicillin, given in a dose of 1·2 mega units weekly for 10 weeks.

Cardiovascular syphilis

It is difficult to assess the benefit of antibiotic therapy in cardiovascular syphilis. If patients survive long enough after treatment, necropsy will reveal that there is a greater amount of fibrosis and relatively less perivascular infiltration of small lymphocytes and plasma cells in the aorta. Prognosis depends more on the general measures taken in the management of the patient's condition than on the administration of antibiotics. There is a strong case for giving penicillin in uncomplicated aortitis in an attempt to arrest the process before the aortic ring and valve cusps become affected, but once aortic incompetence supervenes the prognosis depends on the ability of the heart to compensate for the anatomical defect. Penicillin should also be given to heal other overt or latent syphilitic lesions. As with other types of late syphilis there is no disadvantage in starting treatment with a course of bismuth. Statistically the chance of a Jarisch-Herxheimer reaction causing a rupture of the aorta or complete coronary ostial stenosis is only slight, but when considering an individual patient and his family, statistics might be thought irrelevant. A course of procaine penicillin, 600 mg (1·0 mega unit) daily for 15 to 22 days, is usually considered adequate. Some physicians believe that further penicillin can benefit the patient and give courses, each of ten weekly injections of 1·2 mega units of benzathine penicillin, especially during the winter months. This antibiotic cover does cut down the incidence of intercurrent infections, and gives the physician a chance to keep the patient under closer surveillance during periods when the heart is under greatest strain.

Once the diagnosis of cardiovascular syphilis has been made the physician should discuss with the patient the general measures which will be needed for his care. At the same time he must beware of increasing the anxiety of the patient; in fact he should go out of his way to convince the patient that the prognosis is good, especially if there is no heart failure. A number of patients can worry themselves into an early grave. Nevertheless there will be occasions when the prognosis is grave and a patient will be grateful for the opportunity to put his affairs in order. The patient should normally be advised that henceforward it must be 'moderation in all things', including exercise, diet, alcohol, sex and smoking. If he does not smoke or can give it up, so much the better.

Those with uncomplicated aortitis do not need to change their way of life save in avoiding heavy manual work. Those with angina pectoris will find their own limitations and should be encouraged in the safety of chewing or sucking glyceryl trinitrate (0·5 mg) as often as they need. They should be urged to continue with moderate amounts of exercise while avoiding undue fatigue, as should those with aortic incompetence without evidence of heart failure, although some of them can climb mountains and play sports without any apparent ill-effects. Once there is evidence of heart failure, or if an aneurysm is present, undue exertion should be avoided and a sedentary occupation found. At the onset of left ventricular or congestive failure the patient should be admitted to hospital for assessment. Pulmonary congestion or oedema should be relieved with diuretics, and digitalis treatment started. Adequate sedation is most important at this stage. Nocturnal dyspnoea can be relieved by increasing the number of pillows or by using a back rest. Once the decompensation has been relieved the patient can return home continuing digitalis permanently at a suitable dose. Digitalis toxicity is rare if only given 6 days a week. Diuretics may also be needed from time to time, often when there is an intercurrent infection, each attack of which should be treated vigorously. Medical treatment of aneurysms is restricted to bed rest and adequate sedation, and these measures usually relieve the dyspnoea, cough and pain. Occasionally potassium iodide mixtures give further relief. The results of the surgical treatment of aneurysms and aortic valvular incompetence are rarely as satisfactory in syphilis as in other cases. This is because the surrounding aortic tissues are usually damaged by endarteritis and do not always take the added strain of operation and heal properly. Nevertheless the opinion of a cardio-thoracic surgeon should be sought on all localized aneurysms and those cases of aortic incompetence prior to the onset of failure. Surveillance is for life, and serological findings always take second place to the general health of the patient. It is preferable to examine the patients at three-monthly intervals and useful to have a cardiologist's opinion every year or so.

Neurosyphilis

Penicillin is the drug of choice in the treatment of neurosyphilis and excellent results are obtained in non-parenchymatous neurosyphilis. The usual course is of 600 mg (1·0 mega unit) of procaine penicillin daily for 3 weeks, although some may give a shorter initial course, say for 2 weeks, but follow it with weekly injections of 1·2 mega units of benzathine penicillin for 10 weeks. Retreatment may be necessary in a minority of cases, usually general paresis, when there is clinical progression or the cerebrospinal fluid findings do not revert satisfactorily. Patients with general paresis are prone to Jarisch-Herxheimer reactions which are not suppressed by an introductory course of bismuth. Prednisone, 5 mg four times daily, can be given, unless there are contraindications, for 3 days before starting penicillin, after which it should be tailed off. Paretics may need fairly heavy sedation initially; chlorpromazine, 25 to 50 mg three or four times a day by intramuscular injection or by mouth, is usually effective. In cases of acute mania paraldehyde may be needed. A paraldehyde enema can be given in a dose of 0·5 to 0·6 ml per kg (3 to 4 ml per stone) body weight, or paraldehyde injection, 2 to 8 ml by deep intramuscular injection.

Antibiotic therapy does not carry such a good prognosis in tabes dorsalis, many of the symptoms and signs of which remain unaffected, while the 'lightning' pains may be exacerbated by treatment. Lightning pains should be relieved with soluble aspirin or codeine tablets which may cause peptic ulceration when taken for a long time, or enteric-coated aspirin with paracetamol (Safaprin) tablets which do not cause peptic ulceration. Narcotics are to be avoided as addiction is sure to follow. Lightning pains are often improved by treatment with hydroxocobalamin, 1000 μg daily for a week, then weekly for 10 weeks. Further weekly courses may be needed over the years. Other drugs have also been recommended: phenytoin, 100 mg by mouth three times a day, and carbamazepine, 200 mg by mouth two to four times daily. In cases of intractable pain spino-thalamic tractotomy may be needed. Gastric crises may be very stubborn in their response to treatment. Two ephedrine tablets (60 mg) crushed and taken in water may help, but if the vomiting is severe 0·5 ml of 1:1000 adrenaline hydrochloride by subcutaneous injection may give relief. Occasionally morphine sulphate injection, 10 to 15 mg by subcutaneous injection, may be needed in very severe cases and fluids given intravenously, the stomach contents being aspirated at frequent intervals. Physiotherapy should be given to ataxic patients, who should be instructed in Frenkel's exercises and encouraged to practise them regularly thenceforward. They are probably the most effective form of therapy for tabetics as they keep the patient mobile, muscular tone is maintained and the circulation of the legs improved. Many tabetics complain of poor circulation, with cold feet and muscular cramps. The longer and more woollen the underwear, the warmer the feet and hands become, fashion permitting. An atonic bladder warrants the closest supervision by the physician. Whenever the urine becomes infected the appropriate antibiotic should be given to cure it, but it is important to establish regular voiding of urine, on rising and every 3 hours thereafter until retiring to bed, even though there may be no desire to micturate. This bladder drill also includes the patient pressing suprapubically each time to try to empty the bladder completely; initially this may be helped by giving carbachol, 0·25 mg by subcutaneous injection. Retention of urine may require catheterization initially, but rarely recurs once bladder drill is established. When retention recurs persistently a self-retaining catheter may be left in place for a limited time only.

Charcot's joints are best treated without surgical intervention, except in the case of the vertebrae where the cord is liable to compression. Calipers, made of a light metal such as duralumin, with hinges at the knee to allow flexion, and sufficient padding at pressure points to avoid abrasions, will allow mobility. Arthrodesis in semi-flexion is not to be recommended. The operation is rarely successful and when it is the patient has difficulty in sitting comfortably. A trophic perforating ulcer on the sole of the foot requires constant attention to keep it clean until it heals, and this may take some time. Optic atrophy does not always respond to penicillin alone, but the progress of the condition may be arrested if corticosteroids are given. Prednisone, 5 mg orally four times a day, over a period of several months may be of help.

In neurosyphilis the clinical effects of treatment are usually quite rapid and little improvement is found after three months. Cerebrospinal fluid examination should be carried out 6 months after treatment, at one year and then annually for several years.

The only exception to this would be in the case of 'burnt out' tabes dorsalis where the cerebrospinal fluid findings are negative to start with. The cell count, the globulin and protein estimations should all be normal 6 months after treatment; if not, further treatment may be required. The colloidal gold test usually reverts to normal within 2 years, but the reagin tests in the cerebrospinal fluid may take even longer. Attendance for clinical and serological examinations should continue beyond the 5 years annually for life.

Therapeutic paradox

Very occasionally the rapid healing of late syphilitic lesions, with antibiotic therapy, results in exuberant scar tissue formation which can distort neighbouring structures. Patients with hepatic gummas may develop an obstructive jaundice due to contraction of scar tissue, in excess of that which causes hepar lobatum; patients with aortitis may develop angina pectoris if not already present, in which case it becomes worse, from contraction of scars at the coronary ostia. Hydrocephalus may follow if a lesion adjacent to the iter or aqueduct of Sylvius heals with scarring and blocks the flow of cerebrospinal fluid.

FURTHER READING

Dattner, B. & Thomas, E. W. (1944). *The Management of Neurosyphilis.* London: Heinemann.
Kampmeier, R. H. (1946). *Essentials of Syphilology,* 2nd edn. Oxford: Blackwell.
King, A. J. (1965). The treatment of syphilis. *Practitioner,* **195,** 589.
King, A. J. & Nicol, C. (1969). *Venereal Diseases,* 2nd edn. London: Baillière, Tindall & Cassell.
McLachlan, A. E. W. (1947). *Handbook of Diagnosis and Treatment of Venereal Diseases,* 3rd edn. Edinburgh: Livingstone.
Stokes, J. H., Beerman, H. & Ingraham, N. R. (1945). *Modern Clinical Syphilology,* 3rd edn. Philadelphia: Saunders.

9. Congenital Syphilis

Syphilis is transmitted from the mother to the foetus via the placenta. The infection is therefore prenatal rather than congenital, and the mother must always have the disease herself, although she may lack clinical signs. Congenital syphilis is a preventable disease and only occurs when the mother's syphilis is not diagnosed and treated during pregnancy. The incidence of maternal syphilis depends on the prevalence of contagious syphilis in the community, but wherever routine antenatal serological tests for syphilis are carried out the incidence of congenital syphilis falls dramatically. In the past, congenital syphilis tended to be associated with adverse social factors, far more of them being deprived of parental care in childhood than the rest of the community while the illegitimacy rate was twice that of their uninfected siblings. Nowadays it is associated with fecklessness, either of the mother in not attending for antenatal care, or of those who have charge of her care in not taking the appropriate tests.

While pregnancy is good for the prognosis of syphilis in women, syphilis is bad for the prognosis of pregnancy. Without treatment one-third of pregnancies will end in stillbirth or abortion, but not an early miscarriage, one-third will produce congenital syphilitic babies and one-third healthy children. The earlier the maternal infection the greater the risk of congenital syphilis, but when the disease is of some years duration a healthy child can be born between two others with congenital syphilis. A possible explanation for this is that *T. pallida* are present in the blood stream throughout the early contagious stage, after which they may only appear in showers, the intensity of which decrease with time while the intervals between increase. Stillbirths usually occur when the maternal infection is very early and the infecting doses of *T. pallidum* so great that the foetus succumbs; later overtly infected babies will be born but after the first 2 years of the disease a mother will only infect a foetus when there has been a shower of treponemes during the second or third trimester, once the placenta has started functioning. It is most unusual for a woman suffering from untreated congenital syphilis to infect her own child, so-called third generation syphilis. Once a woman has been adequately treated she cannot infect any subsequent foetuses.

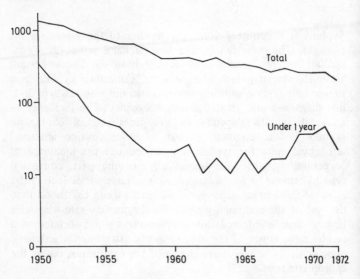

Fig. 8 Congenital syphilis in Britain 1950-1972; total and those aged under 1 year.

A stillborn syphilitic foetus is usually macerated, the skull collapsed and the abdomen protuberant. The skin is a livid red upon which there may be a bullous eruption, the haemorrhagic fluid of which contains many treponemes, as do the enlarged liver and spleen. Neither the appearance nor the histological findings of the placenta can be said to be absolutely typical of syphilis, except on those rare occasions when *T. pallidum* can be identified within it.

The clinical manifestations of congenital syphilis can be divided into an early or infantile contagious stage during the first 2 years of life and a late or tardive and non-contagious stage thereafter, when the stigmata of congenital syphilis are also found.

EARLY CONGENITAL SYPHILIS

At birth a congenital syphilitic baby may appear healthy, lacking any physical signs during the first few weeks. In these circumstances a diagnosis on serological grounds alone should only be made on the results of the FTA-IgM test and possibly by finding that the VDRL test is positive at a higher titre in the baby than in the mother, the titre possibly rising.

Skin lesions. The earliest lesions of congenital syphilis are on the skin. There is no primary sore, the infection being blood borne via the placenta. At birth a symmetrical bullous eruption, 'syphilitic pemphigus', may be found which affects principally the periphery, the palms of the hands and soles of the feet. Treponemata abound in the sero-purulent contents which escape when a bullus bursts. The base of each bullus, upon which a scale or crust may form, is a dull red colour. Within the first month papular or papulo-squamous rashes may develop as in acquired secondary syphilis. They affect mainly the palms, soles, napkin area and around the nose and mouth. In moist areas, they soon become eroded. Condylomata lata often develop at mucocutaneous junctions where, between lesions, the skin becomes 'glazed' in those areas subjected to friction. Radiating fissures may appear at the angles of the mouth, around the nares and anus. With secondary infection they will heal leaving marked radial scars called 'rhagades'. Marasmus, with weight loss and failure to thrive, may give the syphilitic infant an 'old-man look'. The skin is wrinkled and of a yellow-brown tint, 'café au lait'. A syphilitic alopecia may affect the sides and back of the head, or more rarely there may be an abundance of coarse hair on the scalp, the so-called 'syphilitic wig'. The eyelashes and eyebrows may be absent; the nails shed, regrowing irregularly and opaque from a narrow base. The lymphadenopathy associated with the skin rashes may be generalized although often only a few scattered glands can be palpated. When the infection is severe the baby may fail to thrive, have a severe anaemia and succumb to pneumonia or gastroenteritis.

Mucous membrane lesions. Mucous patches occur as in secondary syphilis, in the mouth, throat and larynx. When the larynx is affected the baby develops an aphonic cry. The nasal mucous membrane and underlying periosteum can be involved, causing 'snuffles'. The discharge from this can vary from slight and muco-purulent to copious with blood-stained pus. Destruction of the septum, together with the discharge, may block the nasal passages so that the baby cannot breathe while feeding, causing weight loss.

Visceral lesions. Both the liver and spleen may be enlarged and cause abdominal swellings. The liver damage may cause oedema, due to a decrease of serum albumin with reversal of the albumin: globulin ratio, and a mild icterus. Involvement of the kidneys is mild but some babies do have a slight albuminuria, and a few hyaline or granular casts may be present in the urine. In some early fatal cases a diffuse infiltration of the lungs causes a 'white pneumonia' which will be found at necropsy. Choroiditis is common in the first year, but is difficult to diagnose and usually missed, especially in the absence of other lesions. It is a cause of secondary optic atrophy and its scars later cause the 'salt and pepper' appearance of the fundus. Iritis and interstitial keratitis also occur but are rare.

Meningitis. Mild meningeal involvement is common but is apparent clinically in only about 10 per cent of babies. A stiff neck with a positive Kernig's sign, convulsions, bulging fontanelles, pupillary abnormalities or a hemiplegia may all occur. The cerebrospinal fluid findings are usually either of Grade I or II, but it should be remembered that the presence of reagin in the first eighteen months of life may be due to the normal deficiency of the blood-brain barrier. Untreated early meningitis may rarely cause mental deficiency, hydrocephalus, blindness or convulsions at a later date.

Bone lesions. An osteochondritis, or chondroephysitis, may affect the long bones during the first 3 months of life. *T. pallidum* invades the zone of provisional calcification, which becomes irregular. Granulation tissue is laid down in the region of the metaphysis. This condition is so painful that the infant keeps the limb still, a pseudoparalysis originally described by Parrot. The condition may be complicated by separation of the epiphyses, pathological fractures or a suppurative arthritis. A periostitis may also affect the long bones. Radiologically the epiphysis is seen to be enlarged, the epiphyseal line broad and irregular, the zone of provisional calcification at the distal end of the metaphysis to be thickened, very dense and irregular, giving it a saw-toothed appearance. Decalcification causes irregular patches of loss of density in the bones, especially at the metaphysis. Periostitis of the shaft can be seen together with the subperiosteal deposition of new bone. The upper end of the tibia and the distal ends of the radius and ulna are the sites most commonly affected. The osteochondritis resolves within 6 months, but the periostitis may persist with further layers of bone being laid down in the cortex. During the second year a syphilitic dactylitis may develop. This consists of painless fusiform swellings of the proximal phalanges of one or more fingers or toes, due to a syphilitic osteo-periostitis.

Diagnosis

The diagnosis of early congenital syphilis is made by finding *T. pallidum* in the skin and mucous membrane lesions. The bullous eruption may be confused clinically with scabies, bullous impetigo or a napkin rash, all of which lack *T. pallidum*. The radiological appearances of osteochondritis with periostitis are typical of congenital syphilis, but periostitis alone must be differentiated from a staphylococcal or other periostitis, Caffey's syndrome and double contouring. The serological tests for syphilis are positive, but diagnosis on serological grounds alone needs great care. The presence of specific Ig-M, detected by the FTA-IgM test, is the strongest evidence but a steadily rising titre in the quantitative VDRL test is sufficient. The mother of the baby also must have syphilis.

LATE CONGENITAL SYPHILIS

Any of the conditions found in late acquired syphilis can also be found in the late congenital type, although cardiovascular damage is most rare. Certain lesions, such as interstitial keratitis, eighth nerve deafness and Clutton's joints, are peculiar to congenital syphilis. It is more frequently diagnosed in females than in males, possibly because they are more generally subjected to screening tests for syphilis, as during their antenatal care. About one-quarter of late congenital syphilitics are diagnosed in a stage of latency, although the proportion rises to one-third among family contacts.

Benign tertiary lesions. Benign tertiary lesions are rare under the age of 5 years and over the age of 25. In general, gummatous lesions of the skin and mucous membranes are rare, although they are common in the nose and mouth. Here they are ulcers which perforate the nasal septum causing an irregular collapse of the nose, quite unlike the saddle nose which follows 'snuffles', and of the palate causing regurgitation of food. Lesions of the long bones are usually sclerotic, periostitis of the middle third of the tibia causes the appearance of anterior bowing, a 'sabre tibia'. Localized osteoperiostitis of the skull produces rounded bony swellings in the frontal and parietal areas known as 'Parrot's nodes'.

Neurosyphilis. Between 15 and 20 per cent of patients with late congenital syphilis have neurological involvement although it is latent in about one-third, in which case the cerebrospinal fluid findings are as in acquired syphilis. Vascular lesions are uncommon and usually occur before the age of 10. The onset may be sudden and associated with a severe headache; the effects mild, with isolated cranial nerve palsies or severe, with monoplegia or hemiplegia. The cerebrospinal fluid findings are usually negligible, either Grade I or normal. Juvenile general paresis is rare before the age of 6 or over 14 years. One-quarter of these patients have parents suffering from neurosyphilis. The prognosis is poor and there is a steady and relentless mental deterioration. The cerebrospinal fluid findings are usually Grade III, but may be Grade II. Juvenile tabes dorsalis is uncommon and sometimes runs a relatively benign course. The onset is usually between the age of 10 and 20 years. Among the pupillary abnormalities fixed and dilated pupils are quite common. Optic atrophy is one of the commonest lesions, the prognosis of which is poor. Lightning pains, the various crises, bladder and sensory tract disturbances are all found less commonly than in acquired syphilis, while a positive Romberg test and ataxia are uncommon. The cerebrospinal fluid findings vary from normal to Grade II.

Interstitial keratitis. Congenital syphilis causes a keratitis profunda, the deeper layers of the cornea being affected. This is the commonest lesion in late congenital syphilis, being found in over half of the patients. The initial attack may come as early as in the fourth year or be delayed until the age of 40, but the condition has tended to be relapsing despite adequate, or even super-abundant, penicillin therapy. Usually only one eye is affected initially. The onset is sudden with supra-orbital pain, photophobia, dimness of vision and lachrymation. The process starts as a circumcorneal vascularization of the sclera which extends into the deeper layers of the cornea, where it appears as pink patches. This is followed by an infiltration of lymphocytes. An associated uveitis is usual. Initially there is injection of the sclera with some vascularization of the cornea, possibly only seen by a slit lamp and corneal microscope, but later the pink patches, 'salmon patches', are plain to see. Corneal haze, due to the cellular infiltrations, gives the affected cornea a ground-glass appearance. The keratitis may resolve within three weeks or persist for several months, and is always liable to relapse. Each attack leaves scars, and as these are usually in the centre of the cornea, vision becomes increasingly impaired. In some cases scarring is minimal and vision unaffected, but slit lamp examination will always reveal the 'ghost vessels', empty blood vessels and remnants of the previous vascularization. The finding of spiral organisms in the aqueous humor of patients suffering from interstitial keratitis has cast doubt on its being due to hypersensitivity alone, as had long been thought.

Eighth nerve deafness. A perceptual deafness, due to involvement of the terminal fibres of the eighth cranial nerve in the inner ear, may develop at any age but is found most commonly between the ages of 9 and 15 years. The onset is often with tinnitus and possibly vertigo, followed by the deafness which is usually bilateral. Initially only the higher frequency range is affected, sometimes only detectable by audiometry, but later complete deafness may follow despite intensive penicillin therapy.

Clutton's joints. A painless effusion into the joints, a hydrarthrosis, usually affecting both knee joints and unrelated to trauma, most commonly develops between the ages of 10 and 20 years. Radiologically there is widening of the joint space without any bony change. The condition runs a course of several months, unaffected by penicillin treatment, eventually resolving without leaving any residual damage.

The stigmata. The various stigmata of congenital syphilis result either from the maldevelopment of tissues due to damage caused by *T. pallidum in utero* or soon after birth, or are scars of lesions from both early and late stages. They are to be found in about 40 per cent of patients with late congenital syphilis. The most important are the dental stigmata; maldeveloped permanent teeth which erupt at about the age of 6 years, the central incisors and the lower first molars. 'Hutchinson's incisors' are peg shaped, increased in antero-posterior diameter and with a notch in the narrowed cutting edge. The notch becomes eroded and carious when the enamel is deficient. *Treponema pallidum* damages the central tooth bud which fails to develop, the lateral denticles having to grow inward to fill the gap. 'Moon's molars', or 'mulberry molars' are dome shaped and instead of having four cusps the surface is studded with many small ones. The biting surface is usually deficient in enamel and caries soon supervenes. Maldevelopment of the maxilla with hypoplasia, together with a high arched palate, makes the mandible prominent, causes malocclusion and gives the patient a 'bulldog' jaw. These appearances together with the perplexed expression of those having scars of interstitial keratitis, make up the typical facies of congenital syphilis.

Stigmata due to scarring from early lesions include the 'saddle nose' following snuffles, rhagades around the mouth, nostrils and anus from the early papular rash, and the 'salt and pepper' scars seen on the fundus from choroiditis. Scars of late lesions include those following interstitial keratitis, 'sabre tibia' due to periostitis with anterior bowing, bossing of the frontal bones from healed periosteal nodes, optic atrophy secondary to choroiditis and eighth nerve deafness. Jonathan Hutchinson named a triad of stigmata peculiar to congenital syphilis: the scars of interstitial keratitis, Hutchinson's incisors and eighth nerve deafness.

Congenital syphilis appears to have a detrimental effect, more serious than can be accounted for by its clinical manifestations alone. In the past, about 40 per cent of patients lost at least one term of schooling, but only half of this absenteeism could be attributed to the disease, and then mainly to interstitial keratitis. Many congenital syphilitics appeared to lack initiative, they did not rise in social class compared with their parents, as their uninfected siblings did. They do not tend to be promiscuous nor do they drink to excess, but this may be due in part to a negative attitude to life which is found in many of them. A proportion of congenital syphilitics are actively jealous of their uninfected siblings and deeply resentful of having syphilis through no fault of their own.

Diagnosis

The clinical diagnosis of late congenital syphilis is usually made when one or more of the above lesions are found. The serological findings are as those in late acquired syphilis; the FTA-ABS is always positive, the TPI and VDRL tests usually so while the CWR and RPCFT may be negative. The diagnosis of latent congenital syphilis may have to await the results of family contact-tracing investigations, the mother having syphilis or having been treated for it in the past.

THE MANAGEMENT OF CONGENITAL SYPHILIS

Whenever a diagnosis of congenital syphilis is suspected family contact-tracing procedures should be initiated. In early congenital syphilis the mother will have syphilis and the source of her infection should be sought. It is also advisable to test all the siblings, and the father even if he was not the source. In late congenital syphilis the parents may have been treated after the birth of the patient, but all possibly infected siblings should be tested unless this has already been done.

Penicillin by injection is the drug of choice in the treatment of early congenital syphilis. The recommended total dosage of procaine penicillin is 0·5 mega unit per kg body weight, given by daily injection over 10 days. Occasionally there may be a severe Jarisch-Herxheimer reaction, but in general the prognosis is excellent. The need for retreatment, on the basis of lack of clinical or serological response, is rare but the results equally satisfactory. The reagin tests, the RPCFT and the FTA-IgM test become negative within 6 months while the FTA-ABS and TPI tests may take a year or more. Surveillance should be prolonged and certainly continued into adult life.

The management of late congenital syphilis is as for late acquired syphilis, examination of the cerebrospinal fluid before treatment remaining mandatory. Patients aged 16 or over can be given the full adult schedules, those less than 16 years old only requiring the appropriate proportional dosage. Scars will be prevented if interstitial keratitis is treated immediately with topical corticosteroids, and the pupils kept dilated with homatropine eye drops, B.P.C., to prevent involvement of the iris. Initially one drop every 2 hours of a 0·5 per cent solution of soluble prednisolone is applied to the affected eye, the interval being increased to 4 hours as the inflammatory condition subsides. After several weeks this can be changed to twice daily treatment with 1·0 per cent hydrocortisone ophthalmic ointment, and this may have to be continued for many months. This aspect of the management of interstitial keratitis is best carried out by an ophthalmologist. Penicillin does not enter the aqueous humor as readily as ampicillin, which should be given orally in doses of up to 1·5 g, together with probenecid 0·5 g every 6 hours in a prolonged course of up to seven weeks. Eighth nerve deafness does not respond to penicillin alone, but systemic corticosteroids may be of benefit. Initially 30 mg of prednisone daily, in divided doses, are given for 1 week after which the dose is cut to 20 mg daily for 4 weeks, the daily dose being reduced by 2·5 mg each month as long as the condition progresses satisfactorily clinically and audiometrically. The dose is increased if there is any deterioration.

Surveillance of patients with late congenital syphilis should be continued for life and they should be instructed to reattend immediately they develop any inflammation in the eye.

THE PREVENTION OF CONGENITAL SYPHILIS

Congenital syphilis is a preventable disease, the potential incidence of which varies with the amount of untreated contagious syphilis in the area. It is of the utmost importance, therefore, that all cases of contagious syphilis receive adequate treatment which will render them non-contagious for life. In addition all their sexual contacts must be sought and kept under observation for 3 months from the risk of infection before being dismissed, or if they are found to be infected during observation they must be treated and their sexual contacts sought. A certain amount of syphilis is discovered by means of screening tests for syphilis to which particular groups are subjected. These include, in various parts of the world, blood donors, food handlers, immigrants and those intending marriage. It is very difficult to say what part, if any, these screening tests play in the prevention of congenital syphilis but certainly pregnancy is the most important time for screening tests to be carried out in the prevention of congenital syphilis. Antenatal serological tests for syphilis, which should include a specific test, should be carried out on every woman during the first trimester of each pregnancy, and if possible repeated during the sixth or seventh month. An antenatal test is carried out routinely in clinics attached to hospitals and local health authorities but not by all private practitioners. If maternal syphilis is diagnosed and treated in the first trimester the foetus will not be involved; after that time both mother and foetus are treated. The results of such treatment remain very good, healthy babies being born to women treated in the eighth month of pregnancy. Even though a woman has received adequate treatment for syphilis in the past many would advise insurance courses of penicillin during subsequent pregnancies.

When serological tests have not been done antenatally they should be done at delivery, whether at home or in hospital. If the results are positive inquiry can be made as to possible past and treated syphilis. If this has been adequate the management of the baby is the same as that when the mother has been treated during the pregnancy: namely serological tests taken between 4 and 6 weeks and repeated at 3 months. Antibody and reagin carry over may give positive results at birth and at 1 month but the titre drops with time. When the mother is untreated at delivery and has syphilis, then the baby must be observed, but treatment withheld until a definite diagnosis can be made on clinical, radiological or serological grounds. No harm can be done to a baby suffering from congenital syphilis while awaiting a positive diagnosis. The blind administration of antibiotic therapy to any baby is to be deplored; it does not gain anything for an infected baby but entails years of unnecessary surveillance for the uninfected. Observation up to the age of 3 months with lack of clinical signs and a drop in the titre of the serological tests, ensures that the baby is uninfected.

FURTHER READING

Jeans, P. C. & Cooke, J. V. (1930). *Prepubescent Syphilis.* London: Arnold.

Kampeier, R. H. (1946). *Essentials of Syphilology,* 2nd edn. Oxford: Blackwell.

King, A. & Nicol, C. (1969). *Venereal Diseases,* 2nd edn. London: Baillière, Tindall & Cassell.

Macfarlane, W. V., Johns, H. M. & Schofield, C. B. S. (1955). *The Background of Congenital Syphilis.* Newcastle-upon-Tyne: Department of Venereology, Newcastle General Hospital.

Nabarro, D. (1954). *Congenital Syphilis.* London: Arnold.

Stokes, J. H., Beerman, H. & Ingraham, N. R. (1945). *Modern Clinical Syphilology,* 3rd edn. Philadelphia: Saunders.

10. Gonorrhoea

(Gonorrhoea is a specific and mainly sexually transmitted disease causing septic lesions usually in the genitalia, more rarely in the rectum and occasionally in the mouth.) Non-sexual transmission can cause an ophthalmia neonatorum in babies, a vulvo-vaginitis in young girls and in adults a conjunctivitis by manual contamination or a cervicitis following artificial insemination by a donor (A.I.D.). Metastatic complications affecting the heart, brain, skin and joints are rare. It is one of the most common, if not the commonest, of communicable diseases in the world to-day. The World Health Organization estimated that there were about 150 million cases in 1968.

The causal organism, *Neisseria gonorrhoeae* or the gonococcus, was discovered by Albert Neisser in 1879, although the disease appears to have existed from pre-history. It was probably mentioned in the Old Testament, Leviticus Chap. XV, as a 'running issue (running of the reins) out of the flesh', together with the measures to be taken to prevent contamination of others.

The gonococcus, which cannot survive long outside the body, requires a carbon dioxide fortified atmosphere for culture. It is rapidly killed by drying, heat or soap and water and belongs to the genus *Neisseira* which also includes the meningococcus (*N. meningitidis*) and numerous commensal species, e.g. *N. catarrhalis, N. pharyngis sicca,* etc. The *Neisseriae* are diplococci, the two pathogenic species usually found intracellularly; they are Gram-negative and give a positive reaction in the oxidase test. It is impossible, to distinguish between them morphologically, and although there are colonial differences, they can only be differentiated with certainty by their varied ability to ferment glucose, maltose and sucrose. *Neisseria gonorrhoeae* ferments glucose alone. There are undoubtedly many strains of *N. gonorrhoeae,* some of which can be differentiated one from another by their varying sensitivity or resistance to the antibacterial agents against which they are tested. It is not certain if these strains are pure. Recent work on cultures has shown that there are five serological types of *N. gonorrhoeae* and at least five morphologically characteristic types of colonies. Colonial Types 1 and 2 contain virulent organisms which possess pili or fimbriae radiating from their surfaces. With these they adhere to epithelial cells. The organisms in colonial Types 3 and 4 do not have pili and have lost their virulence. With repeated subculture the proportion of virulent colonies gradually decreases.

PATHOLOGY

Neisseria gonorrhoeae has an affinity for columnar epithelium which it penetrates easily, causing a submucosal inflammation with marked polymorphonuclear response. Stratified and squamous epithelium are more resistant to attack by the gonococcus. In men the urethra, its glands, the prostate, seminal vesicles and epididymes are at special risk, while in women damage is most common in the cervix, Skene's tubules, the few glands lining the urethra, the ducts of Bartholin's glands and the Fallopian tubes. In both sexes the rectal mucosa is susceptible, in women by contamination from vaginal discharges as well as by direct infection as happens in male passive homosexuals. Blood-borne infection from the genitalia occasionally causes metastatic complications, more often in women than in men. The course of untreated gonorrhoea may run for many months, the duration and end results depending on the ability of the patient's body to build up a local tissue immunity to the gonococcus, and to drain away the inflammatory products. Until penicillin was introduced in 1943, sulphonamides never having been effective for long, patients had to cure themselves. This they did with greater or lesser success; many men developed urethral strictures, chronic prostatitis and sterility; women suffered from chronic pelvic sepsis and sterility. Natural immunity, following an attack of gonorrhoea, does not occur, a proportion of patients being reinfected after each cure. The subcutaneous implantation into laboratory animals of hollow polythene spheres, such as practice golf balls, within which *N. gonorrhoeae* can be grown, has opened up the possibility of research into the host factors mediating in gonococcal infections. The vast majority of patients with gonorrhoea produce IgG antibody to the heat-labile surface antigens of the gonococcus and a majority IgA antibodies to the heat-stable somatic antigens, neither of which appears to be protective against future infections. Antibody to the pili of gonococci, which is currently under investigation, appears to block the adhesion of gonococci to epithelial cells within 30 minutes.

EPIDEMIOLOGY

Following the post-war peak in 1946, the incidence of gonorrhoea throughout the world fell until the mid 1950's, since when the incidence has risen to levels in excess of that in 1946 in

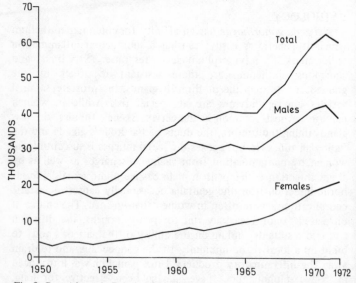

Fig. 9 Gonorrhoea in Britain 1950-1972; total, male, and female cases.

some of the developed and developing countries. The current high incidence throughout the world has given rise to concern because penicillin in sufficient dosage will still cure every infection. The reason for the current rise in incidence has been attributed to many factors, not all of which may affect every area at any one time: the rapid increase in population of many countries after the war; industrialization and consequent urbanization, especially in the developing countries, encouraged the movement of large numbers of single people, including immigrants. In addition, an increasing number of single young people took holidays abroad, using rapid air travel. The diminished sensitivity of an increasing proportion of strains of *N. gonorrhoeae* to penicillin and the other antibiotics in certain areas; the short incubation period of gonorrhoea which hampers attempts to interrupt the chain of infection; the lack of immunity following infection; the high infectivity rate of the disease and the large proportion of asymptomatic women, and to a lesser extent men, especially passive homosexuals; an increase in indiscriminate promiscuity among the young and more sexually active, irrespective of sexuality; the lack of fear of infection, exacerbated by the development of effective contraceptive techniques, and the failure to provide adequate sex education, which appears to be almost universal; all these factors have contributed to the increase in the incidence of gonorrhoea. In countries with an established specialist service, including those of eastern Europe and Britain, the increase has not been as marked as elsewhere.

THE DIAGNOSIS OF GONORRHOEA

Any doctor diagnosing gonorrhoea may be called upon to substantiate it during subsequent divorce proceedings. For this reason, if no other, *N. gonorrhoeae* should always be identified with such certainty that the diagnosis will stand in a court of law. The diagnosis of gonorrhoea is a laboratory procedure, the methods of examination necessary to obtain the appropriate specimens for which having been discussed in chapter 2.

The immediate identification of *N. gonorrhoeae* is usually made by means of Gram-stained smears. Having made a thin smear, or smears, from the discharges or secretions on a clean glass slide, the material is fixed by passing the slide through a flame after which is is allowed to cool. Most specialists use some variation of the Meyrick-Harrison modification of Gram's method. It is most important that the slides are read by someone of experience in order that a correct diagnosis be made at the initial visit, as some patients will fail to return.

Gram's stain

Initially stain with 2 per cent crystal violet for about 30 seconds, pour off the stain and gently wash with tap water; then add Lugol's iodine solution and leave for 30 seconds or less before decolorizing with acetone, pouring it over the material for a few seconds until it runs off almost colourless. Wash the slide in tap water and counterstain with a 2 per cent acid solution of neutral red for about a minute before the final washing with tap water. Blot and dry the slide before examining it under a microscope using a 2 mm objective lens and immersion oil.

Neisseria gonorrhoeae are identified as Gram-negative intracellular diplococci. They appear red, not having taken the violet stain; the diplococci are kidney-shaped, an oval unstained area being left between the adjacent concave aspects; typically they are found clumped within cells. Extracellular Gram-negative diplococci, even though morphologically typical, should not be taken as evidence of gonorrhoea, and even when found intracellularly still require positive indentification by culture. The Gram stain is excellent for recognizing gonococci in the secretions from the male urethra and prostate, but difficulties occur when they are few in number and other organisms are present. This may happen in specimens taken from the rectum, and in the female from both urethra and cervix. *Neisseria gonorrhoeae* must be differentiated from other *Neisseriae,* especially *N. catarrhalis* which is often present in the female genitalia, as are various Gram-negative cocco-bacilli which are also found in the rectum.

Gram-stained smears taken from women at their initial examination fail to reveal *N. gonorrhoeae* in about one-quarter of those suffering from gonorrhoea. When Gram-stained smears have failed to reveal an expected gonorrhoea, duplicate smears, taken at the same time as those used for the Gram's stain, can be used for a direct fluorescent antibody test for *N. gonorrhoeae.* This test will demonstrate the organisms in almost every case, but the technique takes between 15 and 20 minutes to perform.

Rapid direct immunofluorescent test

Very thin smears are spread on a clean glass slide, each within a circle of 1 cm diameter etched with a diamond tipped pencil. The smears are allowed to dry in the air and then fixed by passing through a flame. The stain is prepared by reconstituting with normal saline, rabbit anti-gonococcal serum conjugated with fluorescein isothiocyanate (Difco Laboratories), to which is added, immediately before use, an equal amount of naphthalene black (Messrs Gurr) 1 mg/ml normal saline. A drop of this mixture is spread with a platinum loop over each smear on the slide, which is then incubated in a water saturated atmosphere to prevent drying, at $37°C$ for 8 to 10 minutes. The stain is washed off gently with distilled water for 2 to 3 minutes and the slide dried by blotting and warmth. In some methods the stain is washed off with phosphate buffered saline for 5 to 10 minutes before rinsing in distilled water. The smears are examined using a Gillett and Sibert Conference microscope with a 100 watt quartz lamp emitting ultra-violet light and a dark ground condenser. Sufficient magnification without loss of brilliance, can be obtained by using a X 100 objective lens and a X 6·5 eye-piece. The primary filter is a Turner interference filter (Gillett and Sibert) and the secondary one a Kodak-Wratten 12 gelatin filter. Gonococci appears bright green against a dark red background. Using this technique the only other organism fluorescing at all brightly is *N. meningitidis,* an uncommon inhabitant of the genital tract.

Transport media

The vast majority of cultures for *N. gonorrhoeae* are carried out in bacteriology laboratories. Specimens of pus on dry swabs are only of use provided they arrive at the laboratory before drying out. This may take as little as half-an-hour and rarely more than 2 hours. The development of a transport medium by R. D. Stuart in 1946 opened up the facilities for culture to those specialists working at a distance from a laboratory.

Stuart's medium. Stuart's transport medium and its modifications are non-nutritive and relatively anaerobic preparations of semi-solid buffered agar. *Neisseria gonorrhoeae* survive in its environment which is moist and under conditions of reduction. The medium is usually put up in bijou bottles to which methylene blue has been added. If oxidation occurs the medium turns blue; it is then useless and the bottle should be discarded. Special swabs used for taking the specimens are prepared by being treated with a buffer solution to remove any acid from the wooden sticks and cotton-wool tips, which are then dipped in a suspension of charcoal before drying. These measures were found necessary because acid, and certain batches of agar, are toxic to *N. gonorrhoeae.* These effects are neutralized by using buffered and charcoal-impregnated swabs. The specimen on the swab is plunged deeply into the medium, the stick divided level with the top of the bottle and the cap tightly screwed on. On arrival at the laboratory the swab is used to inoculate various culture media, Stuart's medium being equally effective in holding *T. vaginalis* and *C. albicans* which is a great advantage as they are often present in women with gonorrhoea. Stuart's medium will hold a sufficient number of gonococci for successful culture after 24 hours at normal temperatures or 48 hours under refrigeration, after which times the chances of success are greatly diminished.

Transgrow. The recent development of a selective and nutritive transport medium for *N. gonorrhoeae* and *N. meningitidis* has meant that specimens can now be in transit for up to 96 hours at normal temperatures and the organisms cultured afterwards. It has the added advantage that there is no need to transfer the specimen to another culture plate on arrival at the laboratory. Its disadvantage is that its use is confined to the *Neisseria*. The medium is a modification of the Thayer and Martin selective medium and contains $5 \cdot 0 \, \mu g/ml$ of trimethoprim to suppress *Proteus*; it should be dispensed in 8 ml amounts in flat 20 ml prescription bottles and allowed to solidify as a slope. Before issue an enhanced carbon dioxide atmosphere is introduced which will be retained at inoculation, if the screw cap is only removed briefly while the swab is rolled from side to side over the surface of the agar, the bottle being kept vertical throughout, and the cap screwed back tightly.

The medium can be used in two ways: inoculated bottles can be kept at normal temperatures and sent to the laboratory where they are incubated untouched until colonies develop, often within 24 hours; alternatively the bottles can be incubated for 16 to 18 hours at 34° to 37°C before being put in transit at normal temperatures. Sufficient growth will then have occurred for the *Neisseriae* to survive prolonged transport and the culture will be ready for further examination on arrival at the laboratory. Martin has recently introduced the Gonobag. This is a self-sealing polythene bag containing Thayer and Martin medium in a Petrie dish and a tablet of sodium carbonate. Once the plate has been innoculated the bag is sealed and put in an incubator. Moisture from the warmed medium acts on the tablet producing the enhanced carbon dioxide atmosphere required.

Culture

Immediate culture can be carried out in those departments having an incubator on the premises, the technique is the same as that used in bacteriology laboratories. A specimen from a discharge or secretion is spread with a sterile platinum loop, swab or a charcoal impregnated swab from a bottle of Stuart's medium, over the surface of a warmed plate of an enriched medium such as McLeod's chocolate agar or a selective one such as Thayer and Martin's. This latter medium—which contains 3·0 units of vancomycin, 7·5 μg of colistimethate sodium and 12·5 units of nystatin per ml, and thus suppresses the growth of commensals—should be used for all rectal cultures and whenever there is a mixed flora. The inoculated culture plates are incubated at 35° to 37°C for 24 to 48 hours in a moist atmosphere containing 5 per cent carbon dioxide. The carbon dioxide fortified atmosphere is obtained by using either an air-tight container into which the plates are placed together with a lighted candle or a special container into which a mixture of 10 per cent carbon dioxide in air can be passed from a cylinder. Some colonies will be visible after 24 hours incubation, but the majority take 48 hours. Typically the colonies are discrete, small, circular and translucent, becoming larger, umbilicated and opaque, the margins crenated and the surfaces striated radially and concentrically. When special culture media and lighting systems are used five colonial types can be differentiated. Type 1 are small, dark gold/grey with discrete edges, the refracted components producing pronounced but soft edged highlights; Type 2 are smaller and darker, with very clean cut edges. The surfaces are shiny and the highlights very bright and sharp edged; Type 3 are larger and flatter than Types 1 and 2 and have a dull brown granular appearance. The edges are smooth and lack highlights; Type 4 are smaller than Type 3 but are non-granular and almost colourless, the edges lacking highlights. Type 5 are smaller than Type 3 but as shiny as Type 2. The edges are dark brown and coarsely irregular.

Definitive tests

Once the gonococci have been cultured it is possible to carry out the definitive tests necessary to identify the organism specifically. These consist of the oxidase test and the fermentation reactions, apart from the examination of Gram or immuno-fluorescent stained smears, made from the colonies, for diplococci of the typical morphological appearances.

Oxidase test. A platinum loopful of oxidase reagent, a 1 per cent aqueous solution of tetramethyl-*p*-phenylenediamine hydrochloride, is applied to colonies having a typical or suggestive appearance of gonococci. All the *Neisseria* and some vibrios give a strong positive reaction, the colonies turning pink immediately, then rapidly becoming purple. Much slower reactions occur with *Ps. pyocyanea, Mima polymorph* and some diphtheroids. The oxidase test is very useful when there is a mixed culture and the plate overgrown with organisms, but it is not diagnostic of *N. gonorrhoeae.* The reagent is toxic to bacteria and colonies required for further study must be removed to fresh medium rapidly.

Fermentation reactions. Absolute identification is obtained by means of biochemical reactions which depend on the ability of an organism to ferment certain carbohydrates. An oxidase-positive colony is picked off the culture plate and rapidly transferred to tubes containing 1 per cent glucose, maltose or sucrose, in hydrocele agar. These slopes are coloured red by an indicator phenol red. When the tubes have been incubated for 24 hours, fermentation, and acid formation are indicated by a change in colour from red to yellow. *Neisseria gonorrhoeae* ferments glucose alone; *N. meningitidis,* glucose and maltose; *N. catarrhalis* does not ferment any and *N. pharyngis sicca* ferments all three.

Sensitivity tests

The sensitivity to antibacterial agents of all strains of gonococci should be estimated, most certainly of those isolated from cases of apparent treatment failure. Most laboratories report routinely on the sensitivity or resistance to streptomycin, kanamycin, the tetracyclines and sulphonamides, and when necessary to others such as sulphamethoxazole/trimethoprim, using a disc technique. The results from different laboratories are usually comparable as the discs are prepared commercially. The relative sensitivity to penicillin is mainly estimated quantitatively using a tube dilution technique. Strains requiring a minimum inhibitory concentration of penicillin of 0·1 μg/ml or more are regarded as insensitive. It is often difficult to compare the results of one laboratory with those of another, as there is no accepted and standard method of reporting. Some report penicillin dilutions in units/ml, others in μg/ml; nor do they use the same dilution points in their reports, 0·6, 0·3, 0·15 and so on being used by some, 0·5, 0·25, 0·125 etc. by others. Uniformity would be of great benefit and enable comparisons to be made between strains prevalent in different areas.

Serological tests

The gonococcal complement fixation test (G.C.F.T.) uses a

standard gonococcal antigen and tests for the presence of antibody in the serum. It is rarely positive in early cases of gonorrhoea. In infections of some duration it may become positive, but biological false positive reactions, without apparent reason, are so common among uninfected people that the results of the test are without any diagnostic significance whatsoever. The treatment of patients, especially pregnant women, solely on the basis of a positive G.C.F.T., sometimes done as a routine screening test, is to be deprecated. The diagnosis of gonorrhoea always depends on the isolation and identification of *N. gonorrhoeae*.

Complement fixation, microflocculation and haemagglutination tests are under development which do hold out hope for a specific serological test for gonorrhoea. They become positive early in the disease and revert to negative after cure, but as yet are not sufficiently specific. Cross-reactions have been found with *N. meningitidis*. Specialists would welcome a reliable serological test for gonorrhoea, as a screening test for asymptomatic gonorrhoea and as a confirmatory test when cultures are not available, or have failed to grow. One test, a radioimmune assay for antibody activity to the pili of *N. gonorrhoeae* is currently under investigation and, when developed, may be suitable as a serological screening test. Whilst no antibody can be detected in the first two weeks of the infection, the test is so sensitive that antibody can be detected at levels below 2·5 ng/ml.

FURTHER READING

Amies, C. R. (1967). A modified formula for the preparation of Stuart's Transport Medium. *Canadian Journal of Public Health*, **58**, 296.

Arko, R. J. (1972). Neisseria gonorrhoeae: Experimental infection of laboratory animals. *Science*, **177**, 1200.

Buchanan, T. M., Swanson, J., Holmes, K. K., Kraus, S. J. & Gotschlich, E. C. (1973). *Quantitative determination of antibody to gonococcal pili: Changes in antibody levels with gonococcal infection.* Document of the World Health Organization. VDT/RES/GON/73.79.

Chacko, C. W. & Nair, G. M. (1969). Sero-diagnosis of gonorrhoea with a microprecipitin test using a lipopolysaccharide antigen from *N. gonorrhoeae*. *British Journal of Venereal Diseases*, **45**, 33.

Henderson, R. A., Rutherford, S., Phelps, J. A. & Robertson, P. (1970). Rapid direct immunofluorescent test for the gonococcus as a 'bench' procedure in venereal diseases clinics. *British Journal of Venereal Diseases*, **46**, 205.

Jephcott, A. E. (1972). Preliminary study of colony type stability of *Neisseria gonorrhoeae*, in liquid culture. *British Journal of Venereal Diseases*, **48**, 369.

Kiraly, K. (1973). *Immuno-allergologic aspects of gonorrhoea.* Document of the World Health Organization, VDT/RES/GON/73.81.

Martin, J. E. & Lester, A. (1971). Transgrow, a medium for transport and growth of *Neisseria gonorrhoeae* and *Neisseria meningitidis. H.S.H.M.A. Health Report*, **86**, 30.

Reyn, A. (1969). Recent developments in the laboratory diagnosis of gonococcal infections. *Bulletin of the World Health Organization*, **40**, 245.

Swanson, J. (1972). Studies on gonococcal infection. 2. Freeze-fracture, freeze-etch studies on gonococci. *Journal of Experimental Medicine*, **136**, 1258.

United States Public Health Service (1957). *Gonococcus—Procedures for Isolation and Identification.* U.S. Dept. of Health Education and Welfare, Publ. No. 499.

11. Clinical Aspects of Gonorrhoea

GONORRHOEA IN MALES

The incubation period of gonococcal urethritis is usually about a week, but may be over 1 month. There is often a further delay before the patient seeks treatment of between a day or so and several weeks, depending on the severity of the complaints, so that treatment is often started at least 2 weeks after infection. During this time the patient has remained contagious. Among a series of 231 men attending with gonorrhoea, and not sought as contacts, the average incubation period was 7·9 days. (45·5 per cent developed symptoms in 5 days, 77·5 per cent by the 10th day but 2·2 per cent took over 4 weeks.) The average duration of symptoms was 4·5 days, (in 3 per cent it was over 2 weeks), so the average time from infection to seeking treatment was 12·4 days, although 4·8 per cent only attended 4 or more weeks after infection. Asymptomatic urethral gonorrhoea in males is rare, but presymptomatic infections can be detected by using contact-tracing procedures. When men are sought as the source contacts of women under treatment for gonorrhoea, then up to 40 per cent may be asymptomatic on attendance.

Urethritis

The anterior urethra is the first part of the genito-urinary tract to be affected. Dysuria is commonly the initial symptom, although for the first few hours tingling only may be noted. The burning sensation on micturition is followed by a purulent urethral discharge which may stain the underwear and have an unpleasant odour. On examination of the patient (see chapter 2) there is a purulent yellow or yellowish-green urethral discharge. The lips of the urethral meatus may be oedematous and everted, and a secondary balano-posthitis with a sub-preputial discharge present in the uncircumcised. The source of the discharge can be confirmed by milking the urethra forwards, more pus appearing at the meatus. The two-glass urine test will show a haze of pus cells in the first glass, the urine in the second remaining clear. Complications at this early stage are rare but, as the infection spreads proximally to involve the posterior urethra, they become more common. Some patients claim that after the first few days the discharge becomes thinner and the dysuria less, but the two-glass urine test shows pus in both glasses and 'threads' in the first one at least. Infections are said to be uncomplicated when the urethra alone is involved. Complications occur when the glands and tissues in relation to the anterior and posterior urethra become infected.

Para-urethral ducts. Inflammation of the para-urethral ducts is noted by small beads of pus on either side of the urethral meatus. Untreated they can reinfect the urethral meatus. Chronic inflammation of the ducts may require treatment by cauterization.

Tyson's glands. In Tysonitis pus appears from the para-frenal ducts and may cause inflammation in the neighbouring coronal sulcus. If a duct becomes blocked an abscess will form proximal to, and to one side of, the fraenum.

Littré's glands. Littritis is a common complication of anterior urethritis. There are no special symptoms but it is the cause of 'threads' or 'casts' seen in the urine. Blockage of one of the ducts will cause a follicular abscess.

Peri-urethral abscess. Blockage of a group of ducts from Littré's glands will cause a peri-urethral abscess. If it does not resolve under treatment, the abscess may rupture back into the urethra or, possibly after tracking for some distance within the corpora, through the skin.

Soft infiltrations. When the inflammation has been very severe a 'soft infiltration' of the submucosal tissues may develop around the lacunae of Morgani or Littré's glands. Its presence may only be diagnosed when urethroscopic examination is done as a test of cure or during the investigation of a persistent residual non-specific urethritis following the treatment of gonorrhoea.

Urethral stricture. A stricture due to contractions of scar tissue, may follow either a peri-urethral abscess or a 'soft infiltration'. Strictures can cause difficulty in micturition, a poor and sometimes divided stream of urine or even retention of urine.

Cowper's glands. Involvement of Cowper's glands causes an abscess to form. This may cause dysuria, dyschezia and pain in the perineum. It is a rare cause of acute retention of urine. If untreated the abscess usually ruptures through the perineal skin, but may do so into the urethra or into the rectum causing a proctitis.

The prostate gland. Acute prostatitis causes an exacerbation of the symptoms of urethritis together with perineal and suprapubic discomfort, general malaise and pyrexia. The prostate is found to be tender, swollen and firm if examined, but many physicians would defer such examination until after treatment lest septicaemic complications be caused. A prostatic abscess may form, with symptoms of urgency, terminal dysuria, haematuria, tenesmus and possibly acute retention of urine. Malaise, fever and headache can be quite severe. The prostate is acutely tender and grossly swollen, usually posteriorly; if untreated, the abscess will rupture, and if this occurs into the posterior urethra the patient will experience immediate relief, alternatively rupture into the rectum causes a proctitis; more rarely, the pus may track downwards forming an abscess which opens into the perineum. Resolution of acute inflammation may be followed in the course of time by a chronic prostatitis. Symptoms of this tend to be slight and intermittent, but sometimes persistent; mainly of deep perineal discomfort, worse when the patient has been sitting for any length of time.

Seminal vesicles. The seminal vesicles and the common ejaculatory ducts are often involved together with the prostate. Acute vesiculitis may cause additional symptoms of painful erections and blood-stained ejaculations. The thickened and acutely tender seminal vesicles may be palpated on gentle rectal examination. Incomplete resolution will lead to chronic inflammation, usually in association with chronic prostatitis, while scarring can cause sterility.

Epididymes. Acute gonococcal epididymitis is usually unilateral. The infection reaches the epididymis from the posterior urethra via the vas deferens, and the vas and prostate are also affected. The initial complaint is of pain and tenderness at the lower pole. This pain can increase in intensity to utter agony, the epididymis and spermatic cord becoming hot and swollen, as may also the testis in which case a secondary hydrocele can develop. The patient is pale and ill, with a moderate fever and malaise. If the vas deferens is involved to any extent the abdominal pain may be so acute that appendicitis or peritonitis may be suspected. Abscess formation is very rare indeed, but nodular thickening of the globus minor on resolution is common.

If it is due to scar tissue the lumen will be blocked but there will be no further symptoms; if it is inflammatory, and when drainage of the inflammatory products has been incomplete, it may give rise to chronic intermittent local discomfort. Only rarely are there acute exacerbations with a recurrence of pain, heat, tenderness and swelling. Bilateral epididymitis or recurrent attacks affecting both sides may lead to sterility. Sometimes, when the epididymitis has become established, it is difficult to find *N. gonorrhoeae* in the urethral secretions.

The bladder. An ascending infection from the posterior urethra may involve the trigone of the bladder. Trigonitis causes increased frequency and urgency of micturition with terminal dysuria and haematuria.

Inguinal lymph glands. Inguinal adenitis is found in a proportion of patients with urethritis. The glands are tender and uncomfortable rather than painful. Lymphangitis is rare unless the peri-urethral tissues are affected or there is a marked balanoposthitis.

GONORRHOEA IN FEMALES

Less than 20 per cent of women suffering from gonorrhoea suspect that their symptoms, often trivial, are due to that disease, and then usually from past experience. About one-third of women have no symptoms at all. The incubation period is longer than that for males, usually over 2 weeks, and again there is a further delay before treatment is sought, so that women attending of their own accord are rarely treated within a month of infection. The majority attend as contacts of men already under treatment, and some are referred when a latent infection has been discovered at an antenatal, family planning or 'well woman' clinic and others after they have developed salpingitis or Bartholinitis. As with men they have remained contagious throughout, sometimes reinfecting the source of their infection. The infection is said to be uncomplicated when only the urethra and cervix are affected.

Urethritis

The principal symptom of urethritis is dysuria, sometimes associated with increased frequency of micturition; both are common events in the life of many women and usually 'cured' by a 'bottle of medicine'. The slight urethral discharge is rarely noticed. Examination (see chapter 2) will reveal a yellow purulent urethral discharge, especially if the urethra is milked from above down, and occasionally a red and oedematous urethral meatus.

Cervicitis

Patients with cervicitis may be symptom free, but they may complain of low backache, altered menses when blood clots may be passed and, most commonly, of an offensive vaginal discharge. So many women have these symptoms at one time or another that they do not suspect gonorrhoea as the cause. On examination, and using a Cusco's bi-valve vaginal speculum of the appropriate size, the cervix may appear red or have an acute and angry looking erosion around the os, through which flows a purulent or muco-purulent discharge. Lacking treatment the inflammation becomes chronic, the erosions granular and the discharge less and more mucoid. Naboth's follicles or retention cysts may develop in the cervical glands. Chronic cervicitis has few symptoms, mainly backache, but some women do have persistent dysmenorrhoea and menstrual irregularities.

Skene's tubules. The para-urethral glands may be involved especially if the orifices of their ducts have become patulous. Beads of pus can be milked down the ducts, the orifices of which may be inflamed. Abscess of the glands is very rare.

Bartholin's glands. Infection of a Bartholin's gland causes pain and swelling on one side of the vulva. Walking becomes painful and sitting down uncomfortable. The labium majus on the affected side becomes swollen, red and tender. A bead of pus can be expressed gently from the duct. An abscess forms in the duct when the orifice becomes blocked and eventually this may rupture through the skin or mucous membrane. Untreated Bartholinitis leads to either recurrent subacute attacks or cyst formation.

The bladder. As with other causes of cystitis in women gonorrhoea rarely causes much discomfort, but it does differ in that is rarely spreads to the upper urinary tract. Some women with gonococcal trigonitis complain of increased frequency of micturition and possibly of urgency, but rarely of terminal dysuria and haematuria.

The Fallopian tubes. Gonococci spread from the cervix to the Fallopian tubes causing an acute salpingitis. This may happen especially during the puerperium, after dilatation and curettage of the cervix and in those fitted with an intra-uterine contraceptive device. In the latter two cases it can be prevented by the taking of cervical cultures beforehand. The symptoms of salpingitis may be of acute colicky lower abdominal pains following a menstrual period, with malaise, headache, nausea and vomiting. In some patients the pains are mild but recur over a period of months and may be associated with menorrhagia, dysmenorrhoea and dyspareunia, eventually leading to invalidism, chronic ill-health and sterility. While a patient in an acute attack may appear pale and ill, there is usually only a moderate pyrexia and the tongue is moist. The pulse rate is increased and blood examination shows a polymorphonuclear leucocytosis. Palpation of the abdomen will reveal localized tenderness and possibly a mass in one or both of the iliac fossae. If a pelvic peritonitis has developed there will be muscle guarding in addition. Bimanual examination causes pain on moving the cervix, the 'chandelier' sign, with tenderness in the lateral fornices. A tender fluctuant mass will be palpable if a pyosalpinx has formed. In chronic cases a non-tender hydro-salpinx may be palpated or the cervix and uterus found to be bound down by fibrous tissue, sometimes retroverted and very tender. Acute salpingitis has to be differentiated from acute appendicitis (the most common error), ectopic pregnancy, pyelitis, endometriosis and torsion of an ovarian cyst.

NON-GENITAL INFECTIONS

Proctitis

Gonococcal proctitis in men and women is usually asymptomatic. It is found in over one-third of female patients, usually due to contamination from a copious vaginal discharge, but on occasion is caused by anal coitus, as are all the cases in men. The symptoms and signs are usually milder in women than in men. Women may complain of a rectal discharge or bleeding and possibly of soreness or pain on defaecation. Men may have an acute and deep burning pain within the rectum with tenesmus or, less acutely, a persistent peri-anal irritation or a sensation of moistness. On proctoscopy, the rectal walls of women may appear red and oedematous, but never ulcerated, and are covered with strands of pus or muco-pus. In men the rectal mucosa may be indurated and eroded, the surface more freely covered with pus or muco-pus than in women. With time the rectal inflammation subsides, leaving only a few streaks of muco-pus in the columns of Morgani and occasional patches of mild erythema.

Pharyngitis

Gonococcal pharyngitis is rarely diagnosed or even suspected, but it can occur following oro-genital coitus. There is nothing particular about the pharyngitis or the muco-purulent exudate to connect it with gonorrhoea. The patient may complain of a sore throat and discomfort on swallowing or the condition may lack symptoms and signs. Usually there is some evidence of inflammation, in some cases associated with oedema causing swelling of the pillars of the fauces and uvula or the tonsillar area, and with a slight to moderate muco-purulent exudate. An ulcero-membranous stomatitis has also been reported but the pharyngitis appears to be apyrexial.

Septicaemic lesions

Whenever effective contact tracing facilities are available metastatic complications, due to emboli of *N. gonorrhoeae,* are very rare. The majority of patients are women and while gonococcal dermatitis is a mild complaint the other manifestations are severe and even fatal.

Gonococcal dermatitis. The skin lesions, which are associated with genital gonorrhoea, appear in showers, are scanty and usually peripheral in distribution. Each lesion starts as an erythematous patch which may develop, in turn, into a red papule, a vesicle and pustule, which becomes crusted within a few days, or the patch may be transient. Established lesions are tender, often haemorrhagic and surrounded by an erythematous halo. The oral mucosa may be affected with a stomatitis, palatal petichiae or ulceration of the tongue. The skin lesions are often accompanied by an arthralgia or mild arthritis of large or small joints usually of the upper limb, and when the shoulder is involved a mistaken diagnosis of 'frozen shoulder' may be made. The X-ray appearances of the affected joints is normal. Fever, if present, is mild and intermittent. *Neisseria gonorrhoeae* have been isolated from, or demonstrated in, lesions in the skin, mucous membranes and joints as well as from the blood and the genital tract.

Gonococcal arthritis. Gonococcal arthritis is very rare nowadays and is mainly found in women. To diagnose it gonococci must be isolated from the usually solitary joint affected in the upper limb about one month after infection. It has to be differentiated from Reiter's disease which is much more common in men. The onset is acute with high fever and severe pain on movement of the limb. The joint is swollen and acutely tender, the overlying skin hot and red. Aspiration of the joint produces thick pus from which *N. gonorrhoeae* can be grown on culture. X-ray of the joint shows early destruction of the cartilage and the joint surfaces, with narrowing of the joint space. Without treatment the joint becomes destroyed and ankylosed, the tendons and ligaments around it also being involved.

Gonococcal septicaemia has also been reported as causing meningitis, endocarditis, myocarditis, pericarditis and peri-hepatitis, in some cases fatal. The bacteriological diagnosis is usually unsuspected until cultures from the cerebrospinal fluid or blood have revealed *N. gonorrhoeae*.

Gonococcal conjunctivitis

Gonococcal infection of the conjunctivae of adults or, more rarely in children, is due to manual contamination associated with lack of hygiene. The gonococcal pus originates from the genitalia of the patient, the sexual partner or, in the case of children, a parent. This form of gonorrhoea is extremely rare and usually only one eye is affected. The onset of acute with swelling of the eye-lids, a watery discharge, severe supra-orbital headache, photophobia and chemosis. The discharge soon becomes purulent, the lids stuck together and without treatment the sight can be lost later from corneal ulceration or panophthalmitis. Iritis and iridocyclitis do not occur in gonorrhoea.

GONORRHOEA IN INFANTS AND CHILDREN

Gonococcal ophthalmia neonatorum

Gonorrhoea is one of the causes of ophthalmia neonatorum which, irrespective of its cause is a notifiable disease in Britain. It is defined in law as 'a purulent discharge from the eyes of an infant commencing within 21 days of its birth'. The baby's eyes are infected at birth from the mother's genital gonorrhoea. It is therefore a preventable disease, as is congenital syphilis, but as yet there is no reliable blood test that could be used to screen antenatal women.

Prevention

Some pregnant women develop an offensive vaginal discharge or cystitis. The former is usually due to trichomoniasis or candidosis and the latter to coliform organisms but both can be due to gonorrhoea, which can be masked by the other causes. Full bacteriological investigation and, after the appropriate treatment has been given, repeated cultures to ensure cure and that gonorrhoea has not been masked would reduce the incidence of gonococcal ophthalmia neonatorum. The majority of pregnant women with gonorrhoea have no symptoms, they can only be diagnosed if cultures from the urethra, cervix and possibly the rectum are taken routinely in late pregnancy, preferably at the eighth month. Certain adverse factors may be found in the social background of pregnant women which, when several are present, indicate a liability to gonococcal infection: being unmarried, having previous illegitimate children, being promiscuous or having been treated for gonorrhoea in the recent past, being unco-operative with their antenatal care, the family being on National Assistance or when the husband is away for periods of time. When a number of these factors are present full investigations should be carried out to diagnose or eliminate the possibility of gonorrhoea. If these procedures are carried out antenatal gonorrhoea can be treated in all but the utterly feckless, who spurn all antenatal care and only attend the hospital when in labour. Cultures taken at delivery, however, will be reported upon in time to alert the clinician that the baby is liable to develop gonoccal ophthalmia and not just a 'sticky eye'.

Clinical manifestations

Gonococcal ophthalmia neonatorum usually develops by the fourth day. The affected eye, or eyes, becomes red and inflamed, a watery discharge appears between the swollen lids which become stuck together. Soon the discharge becomes purulent and copious, the conjunctival inflammation and oedema more severe, spreading to the scleral conjunctiva with chemosis. The condition is painful and there is marked photophobia. The pre-auricular lymph glands become enlarged and tender. Without treatment the cornea may become involved with a superficial keratitis, having a ground-glass appearance, later developing into corneal ulcers, which heal with scars causing loss of vision, or even perforation of the globe with loss of sight in that eye. Ophthalmia neonatorum tends to be confused with the ubiquitous 'sticky eye' which is so prevalent in some maternity units and the diagnosis of gonorrhoea delayed by the 'blind' use of chloramphenicol eye-drops. The confusion could be settled if it were agreed that a 'sticky eye' will resolve without the use of antibiotic eye-drops but that ophthalmia neonatorum will not, so that whenever a clinician decides to use local antibiotics, swabs are taken for culture before treatment and the case is notified to the local specialist in community medicine.

Prophylaxis

In the pre-antibiotic era the routine application of one or two drops of 1·0 per cent solution of silver nitrate after swabbing the eyes immediately on delivery, as recommended by Credé, undoubtedly saved the sight of a number of children. Silver nitrate, which is an irritant, was susperseded in some countries by colloidal silver preparations and, when they became available, by local sulphonamides and the various antibiotics. In those countries where antibiotic therapy is readily available, it is doubtful if prophylaxis, or abortive treatment as it should rightly be called, has any place today. Once it develops, gonococcal ophthalmia neonatorum can be cured in every case. No type of eye-drop is 100 per cent successful prophylactically but, when-ever it is, the mother will be left with an undiagnosed, and therefore untreated gonorrhoea. She is liable to develop salpingitis during the puerperium and be a source of infection to others. These health hazards might appear to outweigh any possible good that can accrue to only a proportion of the treated babies. Penicillin, given by injection at birth, is possibly 100 per cent suc-cessful, but the mothers of all the infected babies are left at risk.

Genital infections

Genital gonorrhoea in young boys, which is very rare, is almost always sexually transmitted. The boy may complain of dysuria or his underwear be stained by the discharge and noted by his mother. There are no reports of complications of the urethritis. Sexual assault may result in a gonococcal proctitis which should always be searched for in such cases.

Vulvo-vaginitis

Genital gonorrhoea in young girls causes a vulvo-vaginitis, the vagina being lined with columnar epithelium until puberty. Sexual transmission or assault is the cause of only a minority of cases. It usually occurs when the child sleeps in the same bed as infected parents. In the past epidemics have been reported from various institutions, the infection having been spread by commonly used towels or unsterilized thermometers. The child may complain or soreness or dysuria, or the mother may notice the stained underwear. On examination the vulva is swollen, inflamed and acutely tender. A purulent discharge flows from the vagina and the urethra if it can be seen. An associated proctitis is often present. The diagnosis is made by finding *N. gonorrhoea* in the discharges from vagina, urethra or rectum. Gonorrhoea must be distinguished from the more common causes of vulvo-vaginitis: threadworms and coliform infections from the bowel due to faulty hygiene, sheer lack of cleanliness and foreign bodies inserted into the vagina.

FURTHER READING

Barr, J. & Danielsson, D. (1971). Septic gonococcal dermatitis. *British Medical Journal*, 1, 482.

Catterall, R. D. (1970). The problem of gonorrhoea. *British Journal of Hospital Medicine*, 3, 55.

Iqbal, Y. (1971). Gonococcal tonsillitis. *British Journal of Venereal Diseases*, 47, 144.

King, A. & Nicol, C. (1969). *Venereal Diseases*, 2nd edn. London: Baillière, Tindall & Cassell.

Kushner, I. (1969). Gonococcal arthritis. *Journal of Infectious Diseases*, 120, 387.

Pelouze, P. S. (1939). *Gonorrhoea in Male and Female*. Philadelphia: Saunders.

Rees, E. & Annels, E. H. (1969). Gonococcal salpingitis. *British Journal of Venereal Diseases*, 45, 205.

Thatcher, R. W., McCraney, W. T., Kellogg, D. S. & Whaley, W. H. (1969). Asymptomatic gonorrhoea. *Journal of the American Medical Association*, 210, 315.

Weisner, P. J., Tronca, E., Bonin, P., Pedersen, A. B. H. & Holmes, K. K. (1973). Clinical spectrum of pharyngeal gonococcal infection. *New England Journal of Medicine*, 288, 181.

Wolff, C. B., Goodman, H. V. & Vahrman, J. (1970). Gonorrhoea with skin and joint manifestations. *British Medical Journal*, 2, 271.

12. The Management of Gonorrhoea

Serological tests for syphilis can be taken while waiting for the results of the microscopical examination of the Gram-stained smears with which the presumptive diagnosis of gonorrhoea is made. After treatment, the patient should be interviewed about the source of the infection, if it is not already known, and any subsequent sexual contacts (see chapter 3, Medico-social Management).

Having informed the patient of the contagious nature of the disease, he or she should be advised to avoid sexual intercourse and all alcohol for at least 2 and preferably 4 weeks. The reasons should be given: initially they are contagious and later healing may be delayed or incomplete following the vascular congestion associated with sexual intercourse or the irritant effects of alcohol on the healing urethral walls. Certainly, those men who abstain from alcohol for the first month after treatment have far less chance of developing non-specific urethritis than those who indulge. In addition men should be warned against self-examination, by squeezing the penis looking for further urethral discharge. With regard to their general health, patients should be advised to avoid over-exertion, to take as much rest as possible, to have a bland but nourishing diet and to keep the bowels open. Fluids can be taken liberally but do not influence the prognosis.

The ideal treatment for gonorrhoea is one that can be given with success at one visit. When a course of treatment has to be given over a period of time the patient is liable to default before it is completed, while oral treatment to be carried out by the unsupervised patient, may never be taken as directed. The treatment of an individual patient will vary according to the anatomical diagnosis, complicated gonorrhoea requiring more treatment than uncomplicated; the sex of the patient, women often receiving more than men as the duration of the disease is usually longer and the complications less easy to diagnose clinically; the local resistance or sensitivity of *N. gonorrhoeae* to the antibiotics being used, and this may vary from one time to another.

Penicillin, by injection, remains the drug of choice in the treatment of gonorrhoea, but before giving it the patient should be asked whether he, or she, has had penicillin in any form before, and if so were there any reactions to treatment, e.g. local or generalized swellings, oedema or dermatitis, angioneurotic oedema or anaphylactic reactions. Inquiry should also be made as to any previous allergy: e.g. eczema, asthma, hay-fever. If there has been any previous penicillin reaction its further use is contraindicated; with a history of allergy a patient should only be given penicillin while under immediate observation as an in-patient. To increase the blood levels of penicillin, probenecid, 0·5 g six-hourly by mouth can be used throughout the course.

Several other antimicrobiological agents may be used when penicillin is contraindicated; kanamycin, actinospectacin and possibly cephaloridine by intramuscular injection (streptomycin is not recommended as too many strains are resistant to it); members of the tetracycline group, erythromycin, spiromycin and sulphamethoxazole/trimethoprim orally.

Blunderbuss therapy

Doses in excess of those later recommended in the treatment of gonorrhoea are contraindicated, especially if given over a period of time. If the organism is sensitive the extra treatment is unnecessary and if it is not, the delay in changing to another is unwarranted. The dosage of those drugs which are also treponemacidal should be less than merely suppressive or sufficient to be curative. The larger the number of doses, but not the individual dosage, of an antibiotic (penicillin especially) the greater the chance of an untoward reaction.

Prophylactic or abortive treatment

Treatment without diagnosis is to be avoided whenever and wherever possible, although on occasion the temptations to give it may be great. It is always a violation of that fundamental principle of good medical practice: 'diagnose before treatment'. Prophylactic or abortive treatment should only be given in the case of a woman in late pregnancy, who is a known and accepted contact of a patient with gonorrhoea. To delay treatment in her case may cause an ophthalmia in the baby if she is delivered before treatment, but still full surveillance must be carried out.

Under certain circumstances, when medical and laboratory facilities are inadequate to cope with the number of promiscuous contacts attending for treatment, prophylactic treatment may be the only practicable public health measure possible. It should only be considered a temporary procedure, a stop-gap, until the proper facilities are available. Harm may be done, from the point of view of possible future litigation, when innocent partners receive prophylactic treatment. They may never be able to prove that they had not been infected.

THE TREATMENT OF GONORRHOEA

Males

Uncomplicated gonorrhoea in men is treated with procaine penicillin, with or without probenecid, the dose depending on the sensitivity or otherwise of the strains of *N. gonorrhoeae* in the area. In the United States of America, it is recommended that 1·0 g of probenecid (2 g in Bangkok) is given orally followed half an hour later by the intramuscular injection of 4·8 mega units of procaine penicillin, half the dose into each buttock, or the oral administration of 3·5 g of ampicillin and 1·0 g of probenecid together. In Britain the dose of procaine penicillin given varies from 1·2 to 5 mega units, with or without 0·5 g to 1·0 g of probenecid. Other effective antibiotics include kanamycin 2·0 g by intramuscular injection (the drug of choice for rectal gonorrhoea) and doxycycline hydrochloride 300 mg (three capsules) orally. Local complications are treated by 0·6 to 1·2 mega units of procaine penicillin daily for 5 to 10 days, probenecid 0·5 g often being given orally every six hours throughout the course, or with kanamycin 2 g daily for 3 days or with any of the tetracycline group or erythromycin 500 mg forthwith, then 250 mg six-hourly for 5 to 10 days.

Supportive therapy includes: for severe dysuria potassium citrate with hyoscyamus mixture, B.P.C., 15 to 20 ml, diluted in water, every 4 hours for the first few days; for epididymitis a Scott's dressing (compound mercury ointment) may give ease if applied for 5 days followed by the wearing of a suspensory bandage which can be used from the start if the pain is less severe, from getting out of bed in the morning to retiring at night for at least 3 months. Analgesics, such as soluble codeine or aspirin, or even phenylbutazone by mouth, may relieve the pain, but when it is agonizing pethidine 100 mg intramuscularly or morphine hydrochloride 15 mg subcutaneously may be needed.

Aspiration, using a broad bore needle, or a peri-urethral or Cowper's abscess can be done under local anaesthesia, but excision of any fistula at a later date will require a general anaesthetic.

Relief of acute retention of urine due to a prostatic abscess may be obtained by the use of pethidine or morphine in the dose as above. A catheter should be passed only when absolutely necessary, and not before—and it should be a rubber one. Electro-cauterization of chronically infected peri-urethral ducts or Tyson's glands, under a local anaesthetic, may be necessary. An established stricture will require regular dilatation with either gum elastic or metal bougies up to a diameter of 7·0 mm. There are various scales for the sizes of the bougie but this would be equivalent to number 12 English, 21 Charrière or 42 Guyon. The aim is to dilate the stricture, not to stretch and split the scar which will be followed by further and enhanced scar formation.

Females

Many specialists give more penicillin to women with uncomplicated urethritis and cervicitis than to men with urethritis. In the United States of America the dosage recommended for women is the same as that for men. An initial injection of 1·2 mega units of procaine penicillin may be followed by others on the second or even third day with, or without probenecid. Kanamycin, 2 g intramuscularly, or doxycycline hydrochloride, 300 mg orally, can be used when penicillin is contraindicated. Local complications may be treated with 0·6 to 1·2 mega units of procaine penicillin daily for 5 to 10 days, usually with probenecid, doxycycline hydrochloride 300 mg initially followed by 100 mg twice daily for 5 days, or one of the tetracyclines 500 mg forthwith and then 250 mg six-hourly for 5 days, or kanamycin by injection, 2 g daily for 3 days, especially if there is rectal gonorrhoea. A Bartholin's abscess may need aspiration, sometimes repeatedly, under local anaesthetic with ethyl chloride. With recurrence, excision or 'marsupialization' of the gland may be necessary. Acute salpingitis, with or without pelvic infection, is better treated in hospital. Absolute bed rest and full nursing care are usually needed, the bowels must be opened regularly, the diet kept light and analgesics and sedatives available as required. In the case of acute salpingitis with previous pelvic inflammation an anti-inflammatory agent, such as oxyphenylbutazone, 200 mg three times a day, or a corticosteroid, prednisolone 20 mg daily in divided doses for 1 week, then tailing off, may help in the resolution of the inflammatory process. An abscess may form in the pouch of Douglas; this will need surgical drainage. Chronic pelvic inflammation should be treated with courses of antibiotics in sufficient dosage over a more prolonged period of time, but the prognosis is not always good.

Metastatic complications

If not already in hospital, patients with septicaemic lesions of gonorrhoea should be admitted for complete bed rest and thorough investigations, cultural, haematological and radiological, together with any others considered necessary. In gonococcal dermatitis swabs and cultures should be taken from any skin or mucosal lesions, the genitalia and the fluid aspirated from any affected joints. Gonococcal arthritis is a severe infection; the pus must be aspirated from the affected joint. Very high concentrations of penicillin are required to cure all septicaemic lesions, especially arthritis. Crystalline penicillin 500,000 units by intramuscular injection and probenecid 0·5 g orally should be given six-hourly for up to 14 days, checking by repeated cultures that the organisms have been eliminated from the lesions and by blood examinations that the E.S.R. and white cell count have returned to normal. X-rays should be repeated to evaluate the residual damage. Splinting of the joint may be necessary and to relieve the pain such analgesics as oxyphenylbutazone, 200 mg thrice daily, but pethidine or morphine may be needed initially. Non-weight bearing exercises should be started as soon as possible, initially by passive movements.

Eye lesions. Gonococcal ophthalmia neonatorum and conjunctivitis are treated with systemic penicillin and by penicillin eye drops (10,000 units/ml) two to four-hourly for the first 24 hours, then thrice daily for 3 to 5 days. The systemic treatment for babies should consist of four injections of crystalline penicillin, each of 0·1 mega units, given six-hourly for 3 days: for adults one injection of 1·2 to 1·8 mega units of procaine penicillin, or 2·0 g of kanamycin.

Vulvo-vaginitis. Treatment can be given either by injection of procaine penicillin or by the oral administration of one of the penicillins or the tetracyclines, usually in liquid form. The dose given will depend on the weight and age of the child.

SURVEILLANCE

Males

With effective treatment some symptomatic improvement will occur within 24 hours, there will be less dysuria and frequency, while the urethral discharge should resolve within 48 hours. This is confirmed by the clearing of the urine specimens. Relapse of urethritis due to treatment failure usually occurs during the first week, often without the urine having cleared. It can be caused by an undiscovered complication such as prostatitis, or by organisms resistant to the initial treatment. Cultures should be taken from all cases of relapse as at the initial examination. If an anatomical cause is found it should be treated with the appropriate dosage; otherwise a change in the antibiotic is indicated. Another cause of early relapse or persistence of the urethral discharge is a concommittant non-specific urethritis, with absence of gonococci in the discharge, and this should be treated with a course of tetracyclines. Relapse after the first week may again be due to non-specific urethritis or, if gonococci are present, to a reinfection. This may be from a fresh source or an untreated contact of the initial infection, a so-called 'ping-pong' infection. If there is a fresh source the sensitivity tests may show differences between the old and new strains. In either case a further interview is indicated and the patient retreated.

Once the urine has cleared and remains so, other complications such as prostatitis, have resolved and no further complaints develop, observation is rarely needed beyond the first month. Further surveillance is maintained to eliminate the possibility of a concurrently acquired syphilis. The frequency of examination of the urine varies according to the availability of the patients and the clinical facilities. Usually patients are asked to return twice during the first week; the prostate is examined at one of these visits, and then at weekly intervals for a further three weeks. The observation of patients with gonococcal proctitis is identical, except that rectal cultures are taken each visit.

Some patients default after treatment or when the symptoms subside, and others at intervals throughout surveillance; of those who do keep attending some, if asked to return in 1 week, only do so in 2, and so on. In each case it must be decided whether a patient is more likely to complete the surveillance by continued occasional attendances or, providing they remain symptom free, only attending for the final blood test.

After the first month, at the end of which the serological tests for syphilis should be repeated, attendance is only necessary in the case of reinfection or the development of non-specific urethritis, but many specialists ask patients to attend at intervals up to 3 months from having acquired gonorrhoea when the final blood test is taken before final dismissal as cured.

Females

While post-treatment progress cannot be gauged clinically unless symptoms resolve, it can be judged by the elimination of gonococci from the smears and cultures. In addition, comparison can be made of the pus cell content and type of epithelial cells, surface, intermediate or para-basal, in the post-treatment smears. Although many women claim initially to be symptom free, in retrospect some remember mild symptoms which have resolved with treatment and these patients may become aware of relapse. Relapse due to treatment failure usually occurs within 2 weeks and should be treated by a change of antibiotic. Reinfection can occur at any time, an altered antibiogram often being of help in differentiating reinfection from treatment failures. Reinfection can be treated as was the initial infection.

At each attendance during surveillance smears and cultures should be taken: twice during the first week, then weekly for 3 weeks, arranging that one of them is immediately after a menstrual period. Serological tests for syphilis are repeated about a month after treatment and further smears and cultures are taken after the next two menstrual periods, or over a period of at least 3 months if the patient was treated during pregnancy. Final blood tests are taken before the patient is dismissed as cured.

FURTHER READING

British Co-operative Clinical Group (1971). Survey of gonorrhoea practices in Great Britain. *British Journal of Venereal Diseases,* **47,** 17.

Cobbold, R. J. C., Morrison, G. D., Spitzer, R. J. & Willcox, R. R. (1970).

One-session treatment of gonorrhoea in males with procaine penicillin plus probenecid. *Postgraduate Medicine Journal,* **46,** 142.

Domescik, G., McLone, D. G., Scotti, A. & Mackey, D. M. (1969). Use of a single oral dose of doxycycline monohydrate for treating gonorrhoeal urethritis in men. *Public Health Reports (Washington),* **84,** 182.

Morton, R. S. & Harris, R. J. W. (1974). *Recent Advances in Sexually Transmitted Diseases.* Edinburgh and London: Churchill Livingstone.

Phillips, I., Rimmer, D., Ridley, M., Lynn, R. & Warren, C. (1970). *In-vitro* activity of twelve antibacterial agents against *Neisseria gonorrhoeae. Lancet,* **1,** 263.

Reyn, A. (1969). Antibiotic sensitivity of gonococcal strains isolated in the South-East Asia and Western Pacific Regions in 1961-68. *Bulletin of the World Health Organization,* **40,** 257.

Schofield, C. B. S., Masterton, G., Moffett, M. & McGill, M. I. (1969). The treatment of gonorrhoea in women with sulphmethoxazole/ trimethoprim. *Postgraduate Medical Journal,* **45,** Suppl. (November) p. 18.

Willcox, R. R. (1970). A survey of the problems in the antibiotic treatment of gonorrhoea, with special reference to South-East Asia. *British Journal of Venereal Diseases,* **46,** 217.

Willcox, R. R. (1970). Rolitetracycline by injection and tetracycline phosphate complex by mouth given in a single session in the treatment of gonorrhoea in males. *Acta dermato-venereologica, Stockholm,* **50,** 154.

13. Trichomoniasis

Trichomoniasis is usually a sexually transmitted disease which is much more often diagnosed in women than in men. It is probably the most common sexually transmitted disease found in women, affecting about 20 per cent during their reproductive years. It causes a vaginitis and cystitis, although a large proportion are asymptomatic. In men it usually causes a urethritis or prostatitis, possibly accounting for up to 15 per cent of cases of non-specific urethritis.

The causal organism, *Trichomonas vaginalis,* was discovered by Donné in 1836 in the genital discharges of both men and women. It is a protozoon belonging to the family *Trichomonadides.* Two other trichomonads infest humans, *T. buccalis* in the mouth and *T. hominis* in the lower gastrointestinal tract, but only *T. vaginalis* infests the genito-urinary tract. The various trichomonads can be differentiated morphologically and by culture. *Trichomonas vaginalis* is a pear-shaped organism between 15 and 30 μm long, having four flagella at its anterior end and an undulating membrane down one side. Within the cytoplasm is a large oval nucleus and, at the base of the flagella, blepharoplasts from which also arise the parabasal body and axostyle, which protrudes beyond the organism posteriorly. Reproduction is by fission, the organism initially becoming larger and circular, the flagella and undulating membrane lying flat along the surface: then either two or four daughter trichomonads are formed which soon become motile. Little is known of the life cycle or metabolism of *T. vaginalis.* With phase-contrast, dark-ground or even direct microscopy the organism can be seen in wet preparations and identified by its characteristic jerking and twisting movements, the thrashing of the flagella and the rippling of the undulating membrane. In fixed specimens *T. vaginalis* may be identified using a Geimsa or Leishman stain, but it is most commonly diagnosed by the Papanicolaou stain, more often even than by wet films or culture. *Trichomonas vaginalis* can be cultured in a laboratory if the specimen is sent in Stuart's transport medium. Johnson and Trussell's cysteine-peptone-liver-mallose (C.P.L.M.) medium is probably better than Feinberg and Whittington's medium which contains proteolysed liver and horse serum with antibiotics. Both media will allow the culture of *T. vaginalis* when microscopy has failed.

AETIOLOGY

As diagnostic and contact-tracing facilities have improved it has become evident that the vast majority of infections in women, and all those in men, are sexually transmitted. The highest incidence of the disease is found during the years of greatest sexual activity and among the promiscuous rather than the continent, but it is also found in post-menopausal women and baby girls. It is said to affect the Negro races more often than the white, but it is not known whether this is due to racial susceptibility or not. Not infrequently it is associated with gonorrhoea in women, and demonstration of the gonococcus may

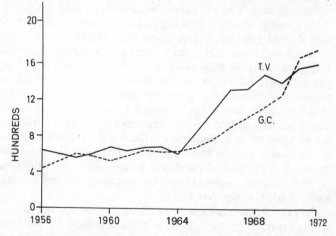

Fig. 10 Female trichomoniasis (T.V.) and gonorrhoea (G.C.) in Scotland, 1956-1972.

be difficult, or impossible, until the trichomoniasis is cured. It is rarely a pure infection, usually being associated with many mixed bacteria and with *C. albicans,* especially if the patient is pregnant or taking one of the contraceptive pills.

The infectivity of *T. vaginalis* is difficult to estimate. In many cases men appear to act as transient 'carriers', getting rid of the organisms completely from the urethra within days; others may remain asymptomatic for long periods, but they can infect women and these do develop symptoms, usually between 1 and 4 weeks after contact. Not all women who harbour *T. vaginalis* develop symptoms immediately; some appear to be healthy for months or years, but they are liable to develop symptoms at any time, especially when pregnant. Non-sexual acquisition of *T. vaginalis* by women has been blamed on lavatory seats, water closets, swimming pools and infected towels. It has also been suggested that female neonates may become infected at birth from their untreated mothers, and the infection lie dormant until adulthood.

CLINICAL MANIFESTATIONS

Women

Many infected women are symptom free; some have a slight vaginal discharge without discomfort and which they can ignore. Others complain of a copious and offensive greenish-yellow vaginal discharge which may cause excoriation of the vulva, perineum and inner thighs, so that sitting is uncomfortable, while walking is agony. In these cases dyspareunia is usual, and this can lead to sexual difficulties, marital disharmony and misery for the patient. When the bladder is affected dysuria and frequency may be severe and acute or occur in bouts, trichomoniasis being one of the causes of recurrent cystitis. The sudden and acute onset may follow upon sexual intercourse for the first time, but the partner is often found to have had intercourse previously. In other cases the onset is insidious, the discharge meagre but worse before the menses, but after a period of months or years dysmenorrhoea and menorrhagia may supervene.

On examination in an acute case the vulva, perineum and patches of the inner thighs are seen to be red and inflamed, some areas weeping when the excoriation is severe. Scars may be present on the inner thighs from previous episodes. If a discharge is present at the introitus it may smell of 'musty hay'. The mucosal surfaces are acutely inflamed and may be oedematous, a purulent urethral discharge appearing at the reddened urethral meatus. Vaginal examination, using a bi-valve speculum, shows a frothy greenish-yellow discharge, which when swabbed away reveals 'strawberry red' inflamed and oedematous vaginal walls and cervix, the cervical discharge being mucoid. In less severe cases the urethra appears normal, although there may be an excess of moisture in the vulva, the vaginitis is mild with only a slight amount of muco-purulent discharge. Sometimes the clinical appearances are normal and trichomoniasis is diagnosed because specimens have been taken from the posterior fornix routinely. Complications include bartholinitis, skenitis, cystitis and rarely pyelitis.

Men

Trichomoniasis in men is usually asymptomatic. Some may have noticed a slight and often transient urethral discharge, possibly only apparent first thing in the morning and associated with localized urethral irritation. When symptoms are mild the patient may not attend until the condition has become chronic, complaining of occasional meatal moisture with mild urethral irritation on occasion, but with long periods of freedom in between. Sometimes the urine is cloudy in the mornings. In more severe cases there is a mild dysuria and some frequency. Occasionally the urethral discharge is frankly purulent, there is discomfort on erection and intercourse is painful. Those who have a long prepuce may have subpreputial irritation and a muco-purulent discharge. On rare occasions the patient may complain of deep seated pelvic discomfort from a prostatitis or even of scrotal pain and swelling due to epididymitis.

On examination inguinal adenitis and epididymitis are rarely found. A balano-posthitis with a subpreputial discharge may be present. While the patient may have a purulent urethral discharge, more commonly no discharge will be seen unless the patient attends in the morning before voiding urine, then a slight mucoid discharge may be found. Usually the urine is clear but contains fine thread, sometimes in sufficient numbers to make the urine appear cloudy. When the second specimen in the two-glass urine test is involved, gentle examination of the prostate should be carried out to see if it is inflamed. If it is, the prostatic bead will contain some pus.

DIAGNOSIS

In women the most fruitful source of trichomonads is the vaginal pool, found in the posterior fornix when the patient is in the lithotomy position. *Trichomonas vaginalis* can also be found in specimens taken from the vulva, urethra or cervix, but not with such frequency. In men wet films are prepared from the urethral discharge, preferably taken before urine is voided in the morning, from the centrifuged deposit of that urine and from the prostatic bead. In the absence of a discharge trichomonads may be found by instilling a few drops of normal saline into the meatus with a pipette, allowing them to flow back and then massaging the urethra forwards, collecting the fluid as it reappears at the meatus. Sub-preputial scrapings should also be examined when there is a balano-posthitis.

The immediate diagnosis of trichomoniasis is made by microscopy. Material from any discharge is obtained on a platinum loop or swab and added to a drop of normal saline on a clean and warm slide, over which a cover slip is lowered carefully to avoid air bubbles. The wet films are best examined by phase-contrast or dark-ground microscopy, using a 2 mm objective lens. Charcoal-impregnated swabs taken from any of these sites and plunged deeply into Stuart's transport medium are sent to the laboratory for culture of *T. vaginalis*. A cervical smear, taken from the rim of the cervical os with an Ayer's spatula, is spread on a slide and fixed immediately with one of the special fixatives. It is allowed to dry in the air before being sent for exfoliative cytology. Trichomonads are found, often in the absence of vaginitis, by this method when the others fail to do so.

Trichomoniasis can only be diagnosed by finding *T. vaginalis,* and with the laboratory facilities available to all doctors in Britain there is no excuse for making a clinical guess. While differential diagnosis does not apply, there are several conditions found in association with trichomoniasis. In women the most common are gonorrhoea and candidosis, which may be masked by it; others include cervical polyps and neoplasms, non-specific cervicitis, senile vaginitis and condylomata acuminata (venereal warts). Trichomoniasis in men may be associated with gonococcal and non-specific urethritis or prostatitis, balanoposthitis due to other organisms, sub-preputial and intra-urethral warts.

THE MANAGEMENT OF TRICHOMONIASIS

Having diagnosed trichomoniasis it is well worth while interviewing the patient concerning any regular sexual contacts who also may be infected. Over a third of them, male and female, will be found to have trichomoniasis, the incidence rising the longer the association and the duration of the infection.

Tinidazole, nimorazole and metronidazole by mouth are all effective in the treatment of trichomoniasis. One gram (two of the 500 mg tablets) of nimorazole taken twelve-hourly for three doses appears just as effective as one 250 mg tablet taken night and morning for 6 days. Two grams (five of the 400 mg tablets) of metronidazole, as a single oral dose, is as efficient as one 200 mg tablet taken after meals three times a day for 7 days. More recently two grams (four of the 500 mg tablets) of tinidazole in a single dose has been shown to give better results than 150 mg three times a day for 5 days. The duration of the courses can be doubled if the initial response is considered unsatisfactory. None of the drugs is associated with toxic effects, though a few patients do complain of mild gastro-intestinal upsets, headaches and skin rashes. Patients on metronidazole should be warned to abstain from alcohol for the duration of the course. On occasions acute confusional states may develop when they are taken together. Patients should be urged to abstain from sexual intercourse until cured. Treatment failure is rarely due to impaired absorption of the drug; usually the patient has failed to take the tablets as directed or has been reinfected, or even both. In the case of reinfection both patient and consort should be treated simultaneously if this was not done initially. Rarely is there need for local treatment, even for women, and certainly never with pessaries which can be most painful to insert. If, however, there is marked vaginal and vulval oedema the application of a 1 per cent solution of gentian violet can be very soothing. When applied liberally it has the added advantage of discouraging some of the infected partners from demanding intercourse before the tissues have healed. Reinfection is much more liable when the vagina is already inflamed.

As with all patients suffering from a sexually transmitted disease, serological tests for syphilis are taken at the first visit, repeated one month later and again before being dismissed. Post-treatment observation of women starts at the end of the course of tablets, when the smears and cultures are repeated, and these should be repeated after the next three menstrual periods. Those who were diagnosed by cytology alone should have repeated cytological examinations to ensure cure. *Neisseria gonorrhoeae* and *C. albicans* will be found in the smears and cultures of a proportion of women after treatment. Surveillance for men is that for gonorrhoea or any other cause of urethritis, prostatitis or balano-posthitis.

FURTHER READING

Catterall, R. D. & Nichol, C. (1969). Transmission of *Trichomonas*. *British Medical Journal*, 1, 765.

Harkness, A. H. (1950). *Non-gonococcal Urethritis.* Edinburgh: Livingstone.

Hess, J. (1969). Review of current methods of the detection of *Trichomonas* in clinical practice. *Journal of Clinical Pathology*, 22, 269.

King, A. & Nicol, C. (1969). *Venereal Diseases*, 2nd edn. London: Baillière, Tindall & Cassell.

McFadzean, J. A., Pugh, I. M., Squires, S. L. & Whelan, J. P. F. (1969). Further observations on strain sensitivity of *Trichomonas vaginalis* to metronidazole. *British Journal of Venereal Diseases*, 45, 161.

Michaels, R. M. (1968). Chemotherapy of trichomoniasis. *Advances in Chemotherapy*, 3, 39.

Ovcinnikov, N. M., Delektorskij, V. V. & Kosmacheva, S. A. (1974). Ultrastructural characteristics of *Trichomonas vaginalis*. An electron microscopical study. *British Journal of Venereal Diseases*, 50, 22.

Robertson, D. H. H., Lumsden, W. H. R., Fraser, K. F., Hosie, D. D. & Moore, D. M. (1969). Simultaneous isolation of *Trichomonas vaginalis* and collection of vaginal exudate. *British Journal of Venereal Diseases*, 45, 42.

Teokharov, B. A. (1969). Non-gonococcal infections of the female genitalia. *British Journal of Venereal Diseases*, 45, 334.

Wallin, J. & Forsgren, A. (1974). Tinidazole—a new preparation for *T. vaginalis* infections. II Clinical evaluation of treatment with a single oral dose. *British Journal of Venereal Diseases*, 50, 148.

14. Genital Candidosis

J. S. Wilkinson, in 1849, was the first to suggest that vaginitis could be caused by a fungus. Yeast infections of the genitalia, which are nearly always caused by *Candida albicans,* have recently been diagnosed with increasing frequency. Genital candidosis, or thrush, is much more often found in women, causing vaginitis and vulvitis. Men may develop balanitis or more rarely urethritis, but are often asymptomatic. It is almost always a sexually transmitted disease in men and often so in women, some of whose infections arise from the bowel. Factors causing the increase in reported genital candidosis include better diagnostic facilities with more widespread use of Stuart's transport medium and the increasing numbers of patients receiving antibiotics, especially those having a broad spectrum of activity, which indiscriminately kill off the bacteria which normally suppress candida.

In general, systemic candidosis is evidence of some severe underlying disease which has lowered the resistance or immunity of the patient. Genital candidosis occurs in association with such conditions as pregnancy, the use of progestogen hormones, diabetes mellitus, pernicious anaemia, the use of immuno-suppressive drugs and the broad-spectrum antibiotics, and in the otherwise healthy sexual partners of such patients. It appears that the vaginal pH is constant for a given woman but it can be lowered by steroids, and when it drops to pH 4, or below, genital candidosis becomes symptomatic.

Candida albicans is the only member of the candida species that is commonly associated with human disease. The organism consists of Gram-positive oval budding yeast-like cells (blastospores), between 3 and 6 μm long, which may form pseudohyphae. These are elongated and filamentous like a mycelium. *C. albicans* is the only species which forms abundant pseudohyphae *in vivo.* The fungus is a common inhabitant of the bowel where it is usually suppressed by the normal bacterial flora.

Its growth is favoured by a change in the bacterial flora, an abundance of carbohydrate and an acid environment. Pregnancy, progestogen hormones and diabetes mellitus are usually associated with superficial infestations affecting the skin and mucous membranes; more severe conditions which lower the patient's resistance, such as malignant disease and organ transplantation, when treated with immunosuppressive drugs and broad-spectrum antibiotics can be associated with systemic candidosis, septicaemia, endocarditis and meningitis.

CLINICAL MANIFESTATIONS

Women

Women with genital candidosis may complain of vulval irritation and a vaginal discharge. The discharge may be copious, white and cheesy or purulent, but most commonly is scanty and watery. It may be minimal while the vulval and vaginal irritation is marked. Excoriation of the perineum and inner thighs is rare unless the candidosis is associated with trichomoniasis, or nylon is worn next to the skin (panties, panti-girdles or tights), which prevents absorption of moisture, or even if a deodorant spray is used which may cause skin sensitization. The infestation is most commonly found in younger women when pregnant or taking one of the contraceptive pills, and in the middle-aged with glycosuria. Many women with genital candidosis have such slight symptoms, or none at all, that for long periods they have no complaints whatsoever. On examination the genitalia may lack signs. On the other hand the vulva may be reddened, swollen and fissured. Some will have vulval erosions or ulcers, and in acute infections the vagina may be so tender that a speculum cannot be introduced. When it can, the vaginal walls are seen to be covered in patches with a sodden and white caseous pseudomembrane, the removal of which leaves reddened haemorrhagic areas. If a discharge is present it is likely to be mucoid or watery, but may have flecks of cheesy material in it.

Men

Genital candidosis in men, when symptomatic, usually causes a balano-posthitis. There is redness and irritation of the glans penis and, in the uncircumcised, of the under-surface of the prepuce. This can vary in intensity from a mild itch to a severe burning sensation. Some men, sexual contacts of women with vaginal candidosis, complain of post-coital irritation of the glans penis. This can be intense and associated with crops of tender vesicles or erosions which heal within a few days. Only occasionally do men complain of a mild urethral discharge, usually worse or only noticeable first thing in the morning. On examination in cases of balano-posthitis the glans penis and prepuce are reddened and tender, the surface covered in patches with crops of vesicles or erosions and adherent plaques of white cheesy material. In some cases, especially in association with diabetes mellitus, the glans penis may be ulcerated and the prepuce oedematous. Without treatment a phimosis will develop together with a watery sub-preputial discharge. The discharge from a urethral candidosis is watery or mucoid and fine specks, rather than threads, are seen in the urine. A number of men, known sources of genital candidosis, have neither symptoms nor signs of urogenital disease by the time they are examined.

DIAGNOSIS

The immediate diagnosis is made by finding large Gram-positive, oval, budding, yeast-like cells, together with the elongated pseudohyphae in vaginal, sub-preputial or urethral secretions, and it is confirmed by culture. Specimens for culture can be sent to a laboratory in Stuart's transport medium or inoculated directly on to Sabouraud's or another such medium. These media are used to confirm that the organism is *C. albicans* by its ability to form chlamydospores. These are large (8 to 12 μm), thick-walled, spherical and refractile cells. All the media have a low nutritive value and a high carbon-nitrogen ratio. Surface-reacting agents are often added to improve the surface spread of the vegetative cells and make the chlamydospores more readily visible. A selective medium, such as potato-carrot-bile, can be used to prevent an exuberant growth of pseudehyphae masking the chlamydospores. When the isolate is predominantly blasto-sporic (yeast-like) on primary culture, another and even more specific test can be used. Cells of *C. albicans* when introduced into serum or other blood derivatives and incubated at 37°C for 1 to 2 hours, will form filamentous outgrowths (pseudo-germ tubes). The appearance of the cylindrical outgrowths, from the previous rounded or oval cells, is diagnostic of *C. albicans*.

As yet the serological diagnosis of genital candidosis is not a practical procedure. Agglutinating and immunofluorescent antibodies are often present in healthy people and may be absent in candidosis; precipitin tests are only positive in association with systemic candidosis.

The diagnosis is based on finding *C. albicans* but the vaginal discharge must be differentiated from that caused by trichomoniasis, gonorrhoea and non-specific cervicitis; the vulval erosions and ulcers from contagious syphilis, herpes simplex and oro-genital aphthosis; the balano-posthitis from that due to trichomoniasis, non-specific infections, balanitis secondary to gonococcal or non-specific urethritis or sensitivity to contraceptives. The urethritis must be distinguished from other causes of non-specific urethritis.

THE MANAGEMENT OF GENITAL CANDIDOSIS

Having diagnosed genital candidosis, and arranged for the sexual contacts to attend for examination, the underlying cause must be sought. In the majority of healthy patients it will be apparent; in women recent antibiotics, pregnancy, one of the contraceptive pills, steroid therapy or diabetes mellitus; in men recent antibiotics, diabetes mellitus or a consort with genital candidosis are the most common causes. If the patients is anaemic pernicious anaemia should be eliminated and if in failing health then a search should be made for malignancy.

None of the antibiotics to which *C. albicans* is sensitive is absorbed is sufficient quantities to allow systemic treatment for genital candidosis. Nystatin is fungicidal and fungistatic, both amphotericin B and natamycin are fungistatic. Vaginal candidosis can be treated with pessaries of nystatin, each 100,000 units, or of amphotericin B, each 50 mg; in either case two pessaries are inserted as high as possible into the vagina at bedtime for 7 to 14 nights. Vulval candidosis responds to either nysatin cream (100,000 units per g), 2·5 per cent amphotericin cream or 2 per cent natamycin cream applied night and morning for 14 days. Natamycin has a cosmetic advantage over the other two in that does not cause any staining. Many infected women also have an infestation of *C. albicans* in the gastro-intestinal tract which is a ready source of reinfection. This can be reduced by the concurrent oral administration of one tablet of nystatin (500,000 units) or amphotericin B (100 mg) four times a day for 1 to 2 weeks. When there is severe inflammatory oedema the initial application of a solution of 1 per cent gentian violet from the cervix to the perineum will give ease.

Candidal balano-posthitis should be treated by washing the genitalia with soap and water, night and morning, and drying them thoroughly with a soft towel, before applying nystatin, amphotericin B or natamycin cream over a period of two weeks. In addition the patient should be instructed to retract the prepuce completely before urinating, after which any drops of urine in the terminal urethra are shaken free before the prepuce is replaced. This helps to keep the sub-preputial sac clean and dry. Urethritis usually responds to daily urethral irrigations for one week of a suspension of nystatin, 100,000 units per ml, or the instillation of phenylmercuric disulphonate urethral jelly on alternate days for 2 weeks. It is difficult to assess the value of treating candidal urethritis as so many cases appear to clear up spontaneously. In some men the post-coital acute balano-posthitis appears to be due to hypersensitivity. *C. albicans* is not found on the glans penis and the men are cured by simple hygiene, providing their sexual partners are adequately treated for candidosis.

Relapse is commonly due to reinfection. In women it may be from the bowel or in both sexes from untreated consorts. In the former case retreatment should include oral treatment and in the latter treatment of the consort as well as the patient. In some cases the infestation appears to be intractable, especially during pregnancy, when repeated courses of oral and local treatment may be necessary. Some patients who are desperate may be cured, when all else fails, by a 28 day course of 2 pessaries (each 200 mg) of povidone iodine each night. In addition, this treatment deals effectively with the offensive smell which so many women find distressing. If the mother is not cured before delivery the baby may develop a thrush of the mouth or genitals. Vaginal candidosis may be as difficult, if not more so, to cure in women taking the contraceptive pills. It may be necessary to change the type of pill or to stop their use for several months, and if candidosis recurs then another form of contraceptive may have to be adopted.

Post-treatment observation is usually carried out for 3 months, smears and cultures being taken at intervals to ensure cure. Serological tests for syphilis are performed as required if there has been any risk of infection within 3 months of treatment.

FURTHER READING

Callomon, F. T. & Wilson, J. F. (1956). *The Nonvenereal Diseases of the Genitals.* Springfield, Illinois: Thomas.

Catterall, R. D. (1971). Influence of gestogenic contraceptive pills on vaginal candidosis. *British Journal of Venereal Diseases, 47*, 45.

Cohen, L. (1969). Influence of pH on vaginal discharges. *British Journal of Venereal Diseases, 45*, 241.

King, A. & Nicol, C. (1969). *Venereal Diseases,* 2nd edn. London: Baillière, Tindall & Cassell.

Lynch, P. J., Minken, W. & Smith, E. B. (1969). Ecology of *Candida albicans* in candidosis of the groin. *Archives of Dermatology, 99*, 154.

Oller, L. Z. (1969). Prevention of post-metronidazole candidosis with amphoteracin B pessaries. *British Journal of Venereal Diseases, 45*, 163.

Winner, H. I. & Henley, R., editors (1966). *Symposium on Candida Infections.* Edinburgh: Livingstone.

15. Non-Specific Urogenital Infections

Apart from gonorrhoea, trichomoniasis and candidosis there are other, often sexually transmitted, causes of urethritis in men, and of cervicitis and urethritis in women, together with proctitis and local complications in both sexes. Metastatic complications also occur, but are found much more often in men than in women. The rising incidence of non-specific urogenital infections now being recognized has followed the more generalized use of cultures which give an accurate diagnosis of gonorrhoea, trichomoniasis and candidosis, and the development of specific and effective treatments for them. Non-infective causes can be found in a small proportion of cases. A discharge may follow self-treatment with antiseptics or even disinfectants; from local trauma, sometimes during coitus; from foreign bodies such as retained tampons; from benign or malignant neoplasms; from scarring or strictures due to previous infections. In all these cases secondary infection by facultative commensals may cause an inflammatory discharge. In addition, infections in the kidneys and bladder may spread to the lower genito-urinary tract. Many organisms have been identified in discharges originating in the genito-urinary tract, some more often than others, but the significance of many of them remains in doubt. A few do appear to produce typical lesions, but they only account for a minority of the cases; in the majority no organisms are found and the aetiology remains idiopathic. As research continues and confirms the specificity of more types of organisms, so the proportion of cases of unknown aetiology, currently over 50 per cent, will drop.

NON-SPECIFIC UROGENITAL INFECTIONS IN MEN

Each year since 1965 in Britain the incidence of non-specific urethritis has been greater than that of gonorrhoea in men, and the gap is steadily widening. Some of the men are contacts of women suffering from trichomoniasis or candidosis, but *T. vaginalis* and *C. albicans* are not always found in their urethral, prostatic or sub-preputial discharges. Some married men deny, no doubt truthfully, that they or their wives have had extra-marital or even pre-marital sexual intercourse.

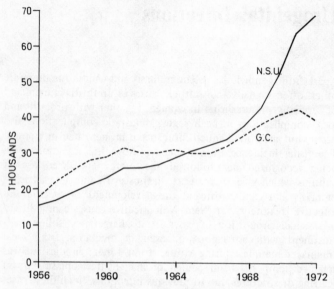

Fig. 11 Male non-specific urethritis and gonorrhoea in Britain, 1956-1972.

Aetiology

Non-infective causes of non-specific urethritis, such as pre-existing strictures, neoplasms, chemical or traumatic inflammations, account for only a very small proportion of the cases seen, as do infections from the kidneys and bladder. Certain bacteria are found in urethral discharges, staphylococci and diphtheroids fairly often, coliform organisms especially in homosexuals and *Corynebacterium vaginale (Haemophilus vaginalis)*. This last organism is not very virulent and in men few organisms are found in the urethra, but the female consorts of such patients often develop a mild vaginitis. *Mycoplasma hominis* and its 'T-strains', those having tiny colonies on culture, are probably commensals. They are ubiquitous, having been found in almost every organ of the body, in sickness and in health. Some organisms found in the urogenital tract may have been acquired orally or nasally, but in the majority of cases the spread is thought to be sexual. The incidence of mycoplasmas within a group may therefore be indicative of their promiscuity, past or present, but no more. *Chlamydia oculogenitale* (Bedsonia) (TRIC-agent), organisms of sub-group A chlamydia are apparently responsible for about 40 per cent of cases of non-specific urethritis, the diagnosis being made by immunofluorescent or Giemsa stains and culture on BHK 21 or Hela cells. They also cause cervicitis in women and inclusion conjunctivitis in the occident. In the orient they cause trachoma and in the tropics lymphogranuloma venereum. Sub-group B organisms cause psittacosis, a disease in humans usually acquired from pet birds such as budgerigars. There is a common blood test for all the chlamydia, the lymphogranuloma venereum complement fixation test (LGVCT), in which an ovine abortion antigen is sometimes used. The blood test only measures group antibody and may be negative in urogenital cases.

Two more sensitive serological tests for *Chlamydia* have been introduced, a radio-isotope precipitation (RIP) test which measures antibody to chlamydial group antigen, as does the LGVCFT, and a micro-immunofluorescence (micro-IF) typing test by which at least thirteen serotypes of subgroup A Chlamydia have so far been identified. The RIP test appears to be the most sensitive one for screening for any chlamydial infection whereas the micro-IF test can differentiate between infection by sub-group A or B *Chlamydia*. Monospecific reactions are more commonly found among trachoma than in urogenital cases, probably because a number of the latter have been infected from several different sources whereas the former would be more likely to be reinfected from within their families.

In those cases of non-specific urethritis in which the pus is sterile it has been suggested that allergy may be the cause: that the male urethra reacts to some allergen in the female genital tract, either a normal secretion or even one altered by the presence of alcohol. So far there is no proof to support this theory, and certainly treatment with corticosteroids or antihistamines neither cures nor prevents non-specific urethritis. The part played by the host has not, as yet, been investigated to any extent. An excess of IgM has been found in the sera of some patients while chromotographic study has revealed an elevated albumin peak and an unknown beta globulin, which is a normal constituent of human urine. These abnormalities were not found in the sera of patients with gonorrhoea or healthy controls. The possibility of some deficiency in the urethral mucosal defence in patients with non-specific urethritis is suggested by the finding that a significantly higher proportion of these patients, than healthy controls, do not secrete ABH blood group substance in the prostatic fluid. In some cases there is dissociation in secretion between saliva and prostatic fluid, ABH substance being secreted in the former but not the latter. In view of the failure to account for every case of non-specific urethritis on an infective basis, the cause may be multifactoral, several of possibly many factors having to be present before the clinical syndrome can develop.

Clinical Manifestations

The onset of urethritis is usually between 1 week and 1 month after intercourse, but may be much longer. Non-specific urethritis may occur coincidently with gonorrhoea, the urethritis persisting unabated after *N. gonorrhoeae* have been eliminated, or may develop following the cure of gonorrhoea. Clinically the urethral discharges cannot be differentiated from one another, but the discharge is often slight and mucoid, worse in the early morning when the meatus may be blocked by the dried overnight secretions, and is not associated with much dysuria. The course of the condition is often relapsing and chronic despite antibiotic treatment. Severe dysuria and haematuria, associated with a urethral discharge, are due to cystitis.

On examination the urethral discharge is usually mucopurulent and rarely copious. It may be absent if the patient has just urinated. Examination is best carried out at least 2 hours after micturition or even before urine has been voided in the morning. An acute meatitis, with papillary congestion or urethral 'follicles' may indicate a chlamydial infection. After taking smears for staining and swabs for culture the patients void urine into two glasses. Fine specks, rather than threads, are usually found in either the first or both specimens, and in the absence of overt discharge the centrifuged deposit can be used for microscopy and culture. Urethral scrapings, taken after micturition, can be used to identify *C. oculogenitale* by smears and culture. Where laboratory facilities are available, a blood specimen should be taken for serological tests for *Chlamydia*.

Local complications

Epididymitis and cystitis are found as often as in gonorrhoea, but prostatitis and urethral strictures are much more common

those without, and if they do so persistently will usually deve
a frank urinary tract infection at a later date. In some cases i
difficult to account for the symptoms, present in the absence
the signs of urethritis but which are usually absent in infecti
such as gonococcal urethritis. Frequency is a symptom
bladder-neck involvement, either from above or below, and
may be that this is caused by either an interstitial cystitis o
urethral infection that lies in the deeper layers of the wall and
presence is not reflected by pus in the lumen, but rather by
desquamation of intermediate and parabasal cells.

Clinical manifestations

The clinical manifestations are much less characteristic than
men. Urethritis, cervicitis and vaginitis, when present, tend to
milder, more chronic and have minimal signs. The contacts
some men with non-specific urethritis lack both symptoms a
signs. Some women with non-specific urogenital infections atte
because they have a vaginal discharge or cystitis. Others
contacts of men with non-specific urethritis and have tricl
moniasis or candidosis with few or no symptoms, but even af
thorough treatment a vaginal discharge may persist. Some of t
contacts have non-specific infections of the cervix alone, b
more often they are associated with urethritis or urethritis alo
is found. Only a few are found to be completely free fro
infection. Cultures from these women with non-specific infe
ions sometimes reveal diphtheroids, coliform organisms or
vaginale. 'Honeymoon' cystitis appears to differ from t
'urethral syndrome'. It is usually caused by an amount of traur
associated with fear and vaginismus on the part of the patier
and lack of technique by the husband, together with possit
secondary infection, but does not tend to recur. Recurre
post-coital cystitis, which may be transient, is associated wi
bacteriuria and may be part of the 'urethral syndrome'.

Some women complain of the recent onset of a vagin
discharge or frequency and dysuria. The cervicitis may be mild
severe and associated with an erosion which may be chroni
Chlamydial cervicitis should be suspected when papillary conges
ion, 'follicles' or nodules together with scars and muco-pus a
seen on the cervix. The vaginal discharge is rarely copious; usual
it is slight and watery or muco-purulent. The urethritis is mil
even with severe symptoms; on occasion all evidence of urethrit
may be lacking.

complications of non-specific urethritis. Non-specific urethritis
may present as an acute haemorrhagic cystitis with, or without, a
urethral discharge. The patient is feverish and ill, and may
complain of passing a few drops of blood after micturition and of
frequency, terminal dysuria and sometimes stranguary. Both the
urine specimens are hazy and flecks of blood may be seen in the
second glass. The urine and any urethral discharge are found to be
sterile on microscopy and culture. Non-specific epididymitis is
usually unilateral and is very difficult to differentiate from that
due to gonorrhoea. In both cases it may follow injudicious
examination of the prostate in the presence of an acute untreated
urethritis and the urethral discharge will have resolved before the
onset of the epididymitis. The patient is usually unwell and may
be feverish, but not as acutely ill as with gonorrhoea. On
examination the epididymis and spermatic cord are swollen and
tender, a secondary hydrocele is often present although the testis
is rarely involved. The condition has to be differentiated from
mumps orchitis, torsion of the testis and epididymitis due to
tuberculosis, as well as from gonorrhoea.

Non-specific prostatitis is often asymptomatic and chronic, in
some cases persisting for years. Only rarely is it associated with
aches or pains in the penis, deep within the perineum, the groins
or in the lower back. Usually it can only be diagnosed by careful
examination of the prostate itself. The gland may appear normal
and non-tender on palpation with a gloved fore-finger, or there
may be areas which are tender and either boggy or indurated. If
the condition has been present for some time, as in association
with recurrent urethritis, the whole gland and the seminal vesicles
may be tender, firm and swollen. The diagnosis of prostatitis is
made by finding an excess of pus cells in the prostatic fluid
obtained by prostatic massage.

Prostatic massage

This consists of gentle but firm pressure with the forefinger
stroking across each lobe from its lateral surface, downwards to
the mid-line; this is repeated three times from either side, after
which the finger is brought firmly down the mid-line to express
the fluid into the urethra. The penile urethra may have to be
milked to obtain the prostatic specimen from the meatus. On
microscopy there are normally no more than two to three pus
cells per 2-mm field of prostatic fluid. In prostatitis at least five,

Local complications

Clinically non-specific proctitis is similar to that of gonorrhoea but, like cystitis, probably occurs more frequently, while the incidence of Bartholinitis and of cysts of Bartholin's glands is about the same. Symptomatically they are usually milder, except when an occasionally severe haemorrhagic cystitis develops suddenly. This is usually associated with fever, malaise, frequency, severe dysuria and sometimes stranguary. The urine is hazy and may contain flecks of blood visible to the naked eye. The incidence of salpingitis is unknown, but is probably far greater than that following cervical gonorrhoea. This is because many attacks of non-specific pelvic inflammation are so mild that they are not diagnosed. Nevertheless the condition appears to be more difficult to treat and relapses are more common, sometimes occurring over a period of years. Sterility can follow bilateral salpingitis, but complete recovery is also known. Recurrent attacks over a period of years are usually associated with a varying amount of ill-health.

The diagnosis of non-specific urogenital infections

The diagnosis of these infections is based principally on the elimination of gonorrhoea, trichomoniasis and candidosis as a cause of the infection by means of wet films, stained smears and cultures. A specific search for *C. oculogenitale* should be made when any lesion in the urethral meatus, rectum or cervix appears 'follicular' or when the patient is a consort of a proven case. Apart from this one positive finding, and possibly the identification of *C. vaginale* or even diphtheroids, the diagnosis of non-specific urogenital infection rests on the finding of apparently sterile discharges.

Differential diagnosis

In both sexes gonorrhoea, trichomoniasis and candidosis must be eliminated. In men the urethritis must be distinguished from an upper urinary-tract infection, possibly associated with calculi in the kidneys or bladder; from urethritis due to chemicals, trauma, urethral strictures, a syphilitic chancre, condylomata acuminata, and herpes simplex infections. In women cervicitis must be differentiated from carcinoma and cervical polyps; vaginitis from that due to foreign bodies and senile vaginitis. Upper urinary-tract infections and herpes simplex infections may be confused with a non-specific urethritis.

The management of non-specific urogenital infections

Men

In the absence of antibiotic treatment the symptoms and signs usually subside within a month or so, in some to recur with complications, usually prostatitis, during the following months or years. As with any urethritis all the patients should be advised to abstain from alcohol and intercourse for at least 2 and preferably 4 weeks. If possible, the regular sexual consort and the source of the infection, if there is one, should attend for examination and treatment.

Penicillin in any form is quite useless in the treatment of non-specific urethritis or its complications. The tetracycline group of antibiotics are the drugs of choice. Uncomplicated urethritis usually responds to tetracycline, 250 to 500 mg every 6 hours by mouth for 3 to 5 days. In practice there is little advantage in prescribing longer courses because so many patients stop taking tablets when the symptoms subside, although some chlamydial infections may need tetracycline for up to 3 weeks; they must be given under supervision. Following treatment with tetracyclines, 500 mg six-hourly for 7 days, recurrence of non-specific urethritis is less frequent when *Chlamydia* have been isolated initially than when they have not. Doxycycline hydrochloride, 300 mg taken with milk in one oral dose is also very effective in uncomplicated urethritis, while streptomycin 1·0 g by intramuscular injection and sulphamethoxypyridazine 0·5 g initially followed by 0·25 g daily for 5 days also gives good results.

Acute prostatitis and epididymitis may need supportive treatment as in gonorrhoea, and tetracycline for 5 to 7 days. Chronic prostatitis is best treated with a course of prostatic massage weekly, or more frequently if necessary to maintain drainage, together with tetracyclines for the first week or two. Soft infiltrations and strictures are treated with bougies, passed at intervals sufficient to keep the urine flowing freely. Dilatation should only stretch the scar tissue and never be sufficient to tear it. Whenever this happens the scar will heal with more fibrosis and further contraction of the lumen.

Post-treatment observation of patients with urethritis is by means of the two-glass urine test, examination of the prostate and prostatic bead, together with serological tests for syphilis up to 3 months, from infection. Chronic or complicated cases are kept under observation until the condition has remained resolved for a sufficient time to ensure that healing has been satisfactory.

Women

The treatment of women is similar to that of men. Usually it is more satisfactory to give partners the same treatment, even in the absence of symptoms and signs, especially if the symptomatic partner has relapsed. As with men, some infections will resolve without treatment, but are liable to relapse, or cause relapses in the consort. Tetracyclines, 250 to 500 mg every 6 hours by mouth for 5 days is usually successful, as is doxycycline 300 mg with milk in one oral dose. Streptomycin and sulphamethoxypyridazine also give good results. Chlamydial infections again should be treated for 3 weeks to ensure resolution.

Bartholinitis and cystitis may require bed rest and one week's tetracycline treatment. A Bartholin's abscess may need aspiration, and a cyst surgical removal. Pelvic inflammations are always best treated in hospital, if the patient can be persuaded to be admitted. Tetracyclines should be given for 1 to 2 weeks, and if the condition is recurrent as gynaecological opinion sought as to possible drainage, or later removal of a chronic hydrosalpynx.

Clinical and bacteriological observation should continue up to three menstrual periods after treatment, serological tests for syphilis being taken before treatment and at 1 and 3 months from infection.

NON-SPECIFIC OPHTHALMIA NEONATORUM

Ophthalmia neonatorum is most commonly due to causes other than gonorrhoea, but in Britain all cases must be notified to the local specialist in community medicine. Many types of organism are found in the babies' conjunctival sacs, including staphylococci, diphtheroids, *C. vaginale* and viruses. They usually cause conjunctivitis within 1 week of birth. Some of these infections have been acquired during delivery from the mother's birth canal, and many of them were originally sexually transmitted. 'Inclusion conjunctivitis', a punctate keratoconjunctivitis due to *C. oculogenitale,* doe not usually develop until the tenth day or later, but can be diagnosed by the usual smears and cultures.

The management of non-specific ophthalmia neonatorum

Most cases of non-specific ophthalmia neonatorum respond to penicillin eye-drops applied every 4 hours until the eye has remained clear for 2 days. Some diphtheroids and chlamydia will require treatment with sulphonamides: 10 per cent sulpha-cetamide sodium eye-drops, and powdered sulphamezathine by mouth, 0·25 g initially followed by 0·125 g every 4 hours are given, again until the condition has been resolved for 2 days. To ensure cure each baby should be kept under clinical and bacteriological observation for at least 6 weeks after treatment.

FURTHER READING

Csonka, G. W., Bassett, E. W. & Furness, G. (1974). Raised serum levels of an unknown beta globulin in the serum of patients with non specific urethritis and Reiter's disease. *British Journal of Venereal Diseases,* **50,** 17.

Dunlop, E. M. C., Hare, M. J., Darougar, S., Jones, B. R. & Rice, N. S. C. (1969). Detection of *Chlamydia* (bedsonia) in certain infections of man—II. Clinical study of genital tract, eye, rectum and other sites of recovery of *Chlamydia. Journal of Infectious Diseases,* **120,** 463.

Dwyer, R. St C, Treharne, J. D., Jones, B. R. & Herring, J. (1972). Chlamydial infection. Results of micro-immunofluorescence tests for the detection of type-specific antibody in certain chlamydial infections. *British Journal of Venereal Diseases,* 48, 452.

Gordon, F. B., Harper, I. A., Quan, A. L., Treharne, J. D., Dwyer, R. St C. & Garland, J. A. (1969). Detection of *Chlamydia* (bedsonia) in certain infections of man—I. Laboratory procedures: comparison of yolk sac and culture for detection and isolation. *Journal of Infectious Diseases,* 120, 451.

Harkness, A. H. (1950). *Non-gonococcal Urethritis.* Edinburgh: Livingstone.

Morrison, A. I. (1969). Non-specific urethritis investigated by Ziehl-Neelsen staining of the urethral discharge. *British Journal of Venereal Diseases,* 45, 55.

Newsam, J. E. & Petrie, J. J. B. (1971). *Urology and Renal Medicine.* Edinburgh: Livingstone.

Oates, J. K. (1969). Prostatitis. *British Journal of Hospital Medicine,* **2,** 556.

O'Grady, F. & Brumfitt, W., editors (1968). *Urinary Tract Infections.* London: Oxford University Press.

Weston, T. E. T. (1965). An allergic basis for non-specific urethritis. *British Journal of Venereal Diseases,* **41,** 107.

Wing, A. J. (1970). Infections of the urinary tract—I. Diagnosis. *British Medical Journal,* **3,** 753.

16. Reiter's Disease

The association between a purulent urethritis, inflammation of the synovial membranes of joints (arthritis) and a purulent ophthalmia (conjunctivitis) in men, was first described by Benjamin Brodie in 1818. The disease, however, takes its name from Hans Reiter who, in 1916, published a case of urethritis, polyarthritis and conjunctivitis following an attack of dysentery, and which he considered to be due to a spirochaetal infection.

In men the arthritis and conjunctivitis or anterior uveitis may follow either sexually transmitted non-specific urethritis or a urethritis which is often asymptomatic, preceded by a dysenteric illness. A dysenteric onset is usual in women; in both sexes it may be a non-specific diarrhoea, amoebic or bacillary dysentery. The sexually transmitted onset is usual in North America and Great Britain, the dysenteric one on the continent of Europe, Asia and North Africa, but irrespective of the mode of onset the subsequent course of events is indistinguishable.

There is difficulty in assessing the true incidence of Reiter's disease as the three main components are not always present in any one form of attack, formes frustes being common, but it probably follows non-specific urethritis in 1 to 3 per cent of cases. The disease is much more common among men than women, the ratio being about 15:1. The first attack of this relapsing condition usually occurs between the ages of 20 and 40, but it is found occasionally in children as well as the elderly.

AETIOLOGY

As yet the aetiology of Reiter's disease is unknown. Its non-gonococcal aetiology has been established for about 30 years, although in some cases the non-specific urethritis is coincidental with or preceded by gonorrhoea, but neither this nor the various dysenteries play any part in the initiation of Reiter's disease. In a few cases the relationship between sexual exposure and the disease appears tenuous, the urethritis even preceding the other manifestations by months or even years. In men damage to the prostate gland appears almost critical; in initial acute attacks the urethritis is complicated, almost always by a prostatitis, and in those cases with a chronic onset or in relapse, by a chronic prostatitis. Certainly a pelvic inflammation appears to be the main provocative factor in men and women.

It is possible that an infective agent, or agents, associated with the urethritis triggers off the development of the other manifestations, the onset of which is not prevented by curing the urethritis. It appears that the necessary damage has been done before the urethritis becomes symptomatic. Of all organisms investigated the *Chlamydia* group seems the most likely to be incriminated, being known pathogens and having been isolated from joint fluid, eyes and genito-urinary tract in cases of Reiter's disease.

In some ways Reiter's disease is similar clinically to rheumatoid arthritis, the type of joint lesions and spondylitis, and to psoriasis, the skin and joint lesions. This raises the possibility that Reiter's disease might be one of a spectrum of diseases including rheumatoid arthritis on the one hand, and arthropathic psoriasis on the other. In the former the trigger may be exogenous (possibly a group A haemolytic streptococcus) and in the latter is probably endogenous. Certainly there is evidence of genetic factors in the aetiology of both diseases and Reiter's disease has been reported occurring in brothers or several members of a family. Investigation of the ABH blood group secreter status in patients with Reiter's disease shows that the vast majority do not secrete ABH blood group substance in their prostatic fluid, but it has not been established whether this is temporary, due to the inflammation, or permanent. The possibility of it being an autoimmune disease has been raised by the finding of antibodies against prostatic antigens in the serum of some patients with Reiter's disease. An increase of lgM has been found during the active stage of the disease, and this is followed by the appearance of an elevated albumin peak. Thereafter, the lgM levels fall to normal and, after a period to time, those of albumin. Chromatographic studies of the sera of patients with Reiter's disease reveals an elevated albumin peak and the presence of an unknown beta globulin, a normal constituent of human urine. The fact that this globulin is also present in the sera of most patients with non-specific urethritis confirms the close relationship between the two conditions. When more is known as to the stages in the disease when the beta globulin is present, then a serological test may become available to confirm clinical diagnoses, especially in atypical cases, and for use in epidemiological studies. The chance that there are many factors and causes in the development of Reiter's disease is even more certain than in non-specific urethritis.

CLINICAL MANIFESTATIONS

The disease may present initially in any one of three ways.

(1) Most commonly an acute non-specific urethritis with a prostatitis, or an acute haemorrhagic cystitis, is followed some days later by a non-suppurative polyarthritis or arthralgia and a conjunctivitis or iritis; occasionally hyperkeratotic lesions appear on the skin and mucous membrane.

(2) A chronic onset with a very mild urethritis, possibly only detected by early morning smears, or an asymptomatic prostatitis alone, the disease presenting clinically with an arthritis or conjunctivitis.

(3) An acute onset with diarrhoea followed after some days or weeks by the other manifestations.

By the time the metastatic lesions have developed there is evidence of constitutional disturbances: malaise, tachycardia (pulse 120 to 150 per minute), a normocytic anaemia with a moderate polymorphonuclear leucocytosis and raised E.S.R. (50 to 100+ in 1 hour). There may be reversal of the albumin: globulin ratio and an increase in alpha-2-globulins. The serological tests for syphilis, rheumatoid arthritis and lupus erythematosus are negative, and the serum uric acid level is normal.

Most commonly the initial attack of Reiter's disease is self-limiting, the urethritis and conjunctivitis clearing within a few weeks, the arthritis taking longer but almost always resolving within a year. Relapses are common, and recurrent arthritis of a joint can lead to permanent deformity while repeated attacks of iritis may lead to blindness.

The genito-urinary tract

An acute haemorrhagic cystitis is the presenting feature in about one-fifth of the acute cases. Acute urethritis is usually associated with an acute prostatitis, although in some cases it appears that an underlying chronic prostatitis has been present for some time. In those cases having a chronic onset prostatic examination will reveal clumping of the pus cells, macroscopically or microscopically, indicating a chronic inflammation. *Chlamydia* or *Mycoplasma* may be cultured from the genito-urinary tract.

The joints

Arthritis is the commonest manifestation of Reiter's disease and is often found in conjunction with urethritis alone. The onset of the initial episode may be acute or gradual, but usually there is a polyarthritis. If only one joint is affected it is usually a knee. Joints are affected in the following order of frequency: knees, ankles, metatarso-phalangeals, less commonly wrists, elbows, tarsals, sacroiliacs and tempero-mandibular joints. In some mild cases there may be no more than an arthralgia. In the first few weeks the arthritis tends to flit from one joint to another; as one improves another becomes involved. When the arthritis is severe the patient is poorly and may appear disproportionately cachectic; muscle wasting of the quadriceps and calves can be very rapid and severe (so-called 'Belsen cases'). The affected joints are tender, swollen and hot. The joint fluid is yellow, turbid and contains numbers of polymorphonuclear leucocytes, a few lymphocytes and occasional macrophages. Culture of the aspirate may be sterile or grow either *Chlamydia* or *Mycoplasmas*.

While the weight-bearing joints in the legs and feet are most commonly affected there may be tenderness over the sacro-iliacs and the posterior spinous processes, with pain on movement. Only occasionally are soft tissues affected, but tenosynovitis of the Archilles tendon and plantar fasciitis do occur.

The initial attack of arthritis usually settles in time, but a few cases do progress to a chronic arthritis. Recurrent attacks of arthritis may be precipitated by sexual intercourse, a recurrence of urethritis or without apparent cause. Relapses may be frequent or at intervals of several years. During relapses there may be widespread involvement of joints or only one, in which case it is usually weight bearing. Some recurrences resolve within 2 or 3 months as completely as the first one, but more often there is progressive joint damage with each attack.

While the knees and ankles may suffer permanent damage the joints most commonly damaged are the sacro-iliacs. A progressive stiffness of the spine develops in almost half the cases which have relapsed. The patients complain of tenderness over the sacro-iliacs, low backache and limitation of movement of the spine, similar to ankylosing spondylitis but less painful. Initially X-rays show blurring of the joint space, later erosions of the bone surfaces and finally obliteration of the joint space. The condition may spread to the lumbar vertebrae with calcification of the intraspinous ligaments.

Repeated attacks of arthritis in the feet may cause persistent pain on weight bearing and difficulty in walking. The commonest cause is a calcaneal spur which follows plantar fasciitis. The typical radiological appearance is of a large and fluffy spur. Less frequently the inferior and posterior surfaces of the os calcis are affected with a periostitis, or a spur may appear at the insertion of the Achilles tendon. Occasionally the only complaint is of pain, localized to the attachment of the plantar fascia to the os calcis, and the X-rays are normal. Some repeated attacks of arthritis leave residual deformities, sometimes a pes planus, but a pes cavus is usually associated with severe damage to the metatarso-phalangeal joints which may result in multiple hammer-toe deformities, with lateral deviation of the toes. X-rays of the metatarso-phalangeal and proximal inter-phalangeal joints show subperiosteal new bone formation, demineralization of the bones with erosions and deformities due to disclocation.

The eyes

Conjunctivitis is found in about half of the cases of Reiter's disease and is usually bilateral. It affects mainly the tarsal conjunctiva of the lower lids at their lateral angles, which become injected, red and covered with a purulent exudate. In many cases the inflammation is transitory but in others it is more severe, spreads to the globe and is associated with chemosis. The condition tends to resolve spontaneously but in severe cases relapses are common. An anterior uveitis may appear during the initial attack of conjunctivitis, but more commonly develops some months after the initial episode and is particularly associated with sacro-iliitis. A chronic prostatitis will be found in men. Anterior uveitis tends to be relapsing and a number of attacks occur over the years, each with painful red eyes and dimness of vision. On examination the sclera is injected, and when the iris is involved synechiae will form which cause irregularity of the pupils. An ophthalmic microscope will show keratitic particles (K.P.) on the posterior corneal surfaces. Each attack tends to cause progressive loss of vision and ultimately can lead to blindness. Other lesions of the eyes are uncommon: involvement of the cornea with either keratitis or ulceration is rare, while optic neuritis, although reported, must be very rare indeed.

Mucous membranes and skin

All the muco-cutaneous lesions of Reiter's disease are associated with hyperkeratosis, their clinical appearances depending upon the type and thickness of the mucous membrane or skin affected.

An erosive balanitis occurs, even in the circumcised, in about a quarter of male patients. The erosions are not indurated but are red and shallow, with slightly raised circinate edges, from which the balanitis gets its name, balanitis circinata. The lesions tend to coalesce as they spread and if dry, to develop keratotic crusts.

Oral lesions can be found in about 15 per cent of cases, but can easily be missed as they are transient, symptomless and superficial. The tongue can be affected with painless erosions or oval areas of reddened papillae. Several types of lesions may be found on the buccal mucosa: transient small opaque vesicles, with surrounding erythema, which develop into erosions; glistening granular erosions with circinate borders which, as they enlarge, become covered with white desquamated epithelium; confluent patches of bright erythema affecting the palate, the tonsillar areas and the uvula, and having a sharply defined anterior border; crops of purpuric spots on the palate.

Skin lesions, affecting mainly the soles of the feet, are found in about 10 per cent of patients with Reiter's disease. The eruption may be generalized in cases of severe arthritis and affect the trunk, limbs and scalp. The lesions start as red macules which develop into vesicles and then pustules which become hyperkeratotic. These fully developed lesions are known as keratoderma blenorrhagica, and histologically are indistinguishable from pustular psoriasis. The heaped-up keratitic material on the surface of the plantar lesions may make them appear like limpets attached to the skin. In some severe cases the nails of the fingers and toes may be affected with a subungual keratosis.

Systemic manifestations

The systemic lesions of Reiter's disease may be very severe

indeed, but are also very rare. There are several types of cardiac lesions, varying from a mild pericarditis to myocarditis with conduction defects, an endocarditis, or even aortic incompetence. They only occur when the disease is relapsing and very chronic. Neurological damage also may occur under similar circumstances and cause peripheral neuritis, including that of the 'shoulder girdle' and meningo-encephalitis. Occasionally the lymph glands may be enlarged and tender, but do not suppurate, while thrombophlebitis has been reported. Gastro-intestinal amyloidosis, as a complication of Reiter's disease, has also been recorded

THE DIAGNOSIS OF REITER'S DISEASE

There is no specific test for Reiter's disease, but the presence of *Chlamydia* in affected eyes and joints as well as in the genito-urinary tract is very suggestive indeed, and a specific search for these organisms should always be made when the diagnosis is in doubt. In typical cases the history and the clinical findings of urethritis, prostatitis, acute haemorrhagic cystitis or dysentery, followed by arthritis and conjunctivitis or iritis, should clinch the diagnosis. In addition the typical radiological appearances of the affected sacro-iliac joints, calcaneal spurs and the other deformities of the feet, the presence of a raised E.S.R. and the elimination of other conditions by means of negative cultures, biochemical and serological tests, should prevent confusion.

Differential diagnosis

Reiter's disease must be distinguished from gonococcal or other infective arthritis, rheumatoid arthritis, ankylosing spondylitis, systemic lupus erythematosus, psoriatic athropathy, gout, rheumatic fever, serum sickness and oro-genital aphthosis.

THE MANAGEMENT OF REITER'S DISEASE

In those cases in which Reiter's disease has followed a sexually transmitted disease serological tests for syphilis should be taken at intervals up to 3 months from risk of infection, and the sexual partners examined.

Treatment of the initial or any acute attack is best carried out in hospital. Certainly bed rest, proper nursing and regular analgesics are required in the treatment of an acute arthritis, while regular physiotherapy is necessary during the recovery period. The diet should be nutritious and varied, and it is worthy of note that a number of patients with Reiter's disease develop a very good appetite, in contrast with other acute arthritic patients.

The urethritis tends to be relapsing and may be resistant to the routine treatment given for non-specific urethritis. Tetracyclines remain the drugs of choice, but the course should be prolonged, especially if *Chlamydia* have been isolated from any of the lesions. Tetracycline, 250 mg every 6 hours, should be given by mouth for 2 to 3 weeks, together with vitamin B (Strong Vitamin B Tables, B.P.C., 1 thrice daily), if there is any bowel upset or proctitis. A prostatitis may need prostatic massage at intervals to maintain drainage of the gland and an acute haemorrhagic cystitis potassium citrate and hyoscyasmus mixture, B.P.C., 15 to 30 ml, diluted in water as required, to suppress severe dysuria or stranguary.

Arthritis, when mild, or arthralgia may respond to bed rest and soluble aspirin alone. In more severe cases the joint, or joints, may need the application of a firm pressure bandage during the day and support with light splints at night, while aspiration of some of the joint fluid may be needed if the synovia is tense, together with stronger analgesics. A number of suitable analgesics are available: indomethacin, one 25 mg capsule three times a day with food, increasing each individual dose to a 50 mg capsule if necessary, is usually very effective. At night, or in the presence of gastric upsets, one 100 mg suppository can be used. Tablets of either phenylbutazone or oxyphenylbutazone, 200 mg three times a day, are also effective, but a watch should be kept for the possible development of blood dyscrasias. The use of cytotoxic or immunosuppressive drugs is rarely warranted, and then only when the clinical condition deteriorates despite active therapy. Pain in the insertion of the Achilles tendon or in the plantar fascia may be relieved by infiltration with corticosteroids.

Intra-articular injection may also ease persistent pain, but their use is fraught with danger, not the least being the development of a Charcot joint if weight bearing is permitted. Methotrexate, 25 mg by mouth weekly for 2 to 3 months, or prednisone, initially 60 mg daily by mouth and in divided doses, reducing to a maintenance dose of 15 to 30 mg daily for at least 3 months, may be effective when other measures have failed, but the condition is liable to relapse once the treatment is stopped.

Conjunctivitis rarely needs local treatment. When severe it can be arrested by using 0·5 per cent prednisolone sodium phosphate eye-drops, B.P.C., three times a day. The management of anterior uveitis is best carried out in collaboration with an ophthalmologist. The pupils should be kept dilated with homatropine eye-drops, B.P.C., and the inflammation suppressed with a topical cortico-steroid such as prednisolone eye-drops. Only very occasionally are systemic corticosteroids indicated, and then in doses as for arthritis.

Mouth lesions do not require any treatment. Balanitis circinata may resolve more rapidly if treated with a cream or ointment containing 1·0 per cent of hydrocortisone and 0·5 per cent of kanamycin. Keratoderma blenorrhagica sometimes improves when treated with a cream containing either 0·1 per cent triamcinolone acetonide or 0·2 per cent fluocinolone acetonide under an occlusive dressing.

The more serious systemic manifestations of Reiter's disease, including the cardiac and neurological lesions, usually require systemic corticosteroid therapy. Such cases are better managed in collaboration with a physician having a special interest in that particular field of medicine.

In view of the relapsing and chronic nature of Reiter's disease, follow up, subsequent to treatment, should be prolonged for several years. Patients should attend for regular examinations to exclude the recurrence of prostatitis and to ensure that such conditions as sacro-iliitis do not develop or progress. All patients treated for Reiter's disease should be advised to return whenever they have any complaints concerning their eyes, joints or genito-urinary tract.

FURTHER READING

Brodie, B. (1836). *Pathological and Surgical Observations on Diseases of the Joints,* 4th edn. London: Longman, Hurst, Rees, Orme & Brown.

Catterall, R. D., Rooney, K. J. & Kirby, B. (1965). Neuralgic amyotrophy in Reiter's disease. *British Journal of Venereal Diseases,* 41, 62.

Copeman, W. S. C. editor (1968). *Textbook of Rheumatic Diseases.* Edinburgh: Livingstone.

Csonka, G. W., Litchfield, J. W., Oates, J. K. & Willcox, R. R. (1961). Cardiac lesions in Reiter's disease. *British Medical Journal,* 1, 243.

Dryll, A., Kaln, M. F., Solnica, J., Mitrovis, D. & Sèze, S. de (1969). Overlapping forms of Reiter's syndrome and psoriatic arthropathy. *Semaine des Hôpitaux de Paris,* 45, 499.

Hancock, J. A. H. (1965). Reiter's disease. *Practitioner,* 195, 605.

King, A. J. & Nicol, C. (1969). *Venereal Diseases,* 2nd edn. London: Baillière, Tindall & Cassell.

Morton, R. S. & Harris, R. J. W. (1974). *Recent Advances in Sexually Transmitted Diseases*. Edinburgh and London: Churchill Livingstone.
Sairanen, E., Paronen, I. & Mähönen, H. (1969). Reiter's syndrome; a follow-up study. *Acta medica scandinavica*, **185**, 57.

the penis; in women, on the vulva, the walls of the vagina and the cervix. In women spread to the perineum and peri-anal area does occur from vulval lesions, but in men peri-anal and rectal warts are mainly found among homosexuals.

A genital wart usually starts as a red or pink pin-head sized swelling which grows upward and becomes pedunculated. It is usually surrounded by similar protuberances which ultimately give the lesion a cauliflower appearance. This may vary in size from a few millimetres to 10 cm or more, peri-anal lesions usually being the largest. On occasions there is extensive spread of warts in the locality of the original lesion. Individual warts tend to develop rapidly during pregnancy; otherwise their growth is enhanced when they are in moist or wet surroundings, as in the presence of a persistent discharge, or when personal hygiene is poor.

Condylomata acuminata must be distinguished from condylomata lata, the warty growths of secondary syphilis. This can be done by dark-ground examination of scrapings taken from the lesions. When a wart is large it must be differentiated from a fungating carcinoma by biopsy.

Management

Sexual contacts should be examined whenever possible. In practice this usually means the regular consort only, as the source of the infection, possibly of 6 or more months duration, is usually unknown. Serological tests for syphilis should be carried out on the patient initially and up to 3 months from infection. The successful treatment of genital warts depends on the maintenance of strict personal hygiene, and the elimination of any discharges present. In women genital warts are often associated with trichomoniasis or vaginal candidosis, and will not respond to any treatment until that infection is cured. Warts on the mucous membranes sometimes respond to the application of trichloracetic acid or 20 per cent podophyllin. If the vehicle is alcohol or compound benzoin tincture care must be taken to avoid contamination of the surrounding tissues lest the podophyllin causes ulcers. Using liquid paraffin as a vehicle there is less chance of local damage, but the treated parts should be washed clean 2 to 4 hours afterwards as for the other forms of treatment. Podophyllin needs to be applied several times a week, if possible, until the warts are cleared. A more effective treatment has been introduced recently. Cryosurgery, with an instrument such as the Dynatech Model DCG-800 Dynagyne, using nitrous oxide, freezes the wart to $-70°C$. The careful application of K-Y lubricating jelly to the wart alone ensures a good and painless contact. No more than 2 to 3 treatment sessions are required if the instrument is applied to each part of the wart for periods of about one minute. Forty per cent idoxuridine in DMSO for 4 days has not proved to be so successful.

MOLLUSCUM CONTAGIOSUM

Molluscum contagiosum is a contagious disease which affects the skin rather than the mucous membranes and may be transmitted in swimming or Turkish baths or by close bodily contact, including sexual intercourse. The causal organism is a virus, the largest of the pox-viruses known to be pathogenic to man. The hemispherical papular lesions are so superficial that there is insufficient contact between the host and virus to produce antibody. The papules vary in the size from 1 to 5 mm, are waxy and white to pale pink in colour. Characteristically there is a central depression which may be filled with a white plug. The contents of mature papules is a semi-solid, white and sticky mass which, if spread on a slide and stained by Giemsa's method, is shown to include many large ballooned cells containing inclusion bodies.

In an atopic subject the papules may be widely distributed. With an asexual transmission they are usually found on the trunk and limbs. As a sexually transmitted disease the lesions are confined to the genital area, on the thighs in both sexes, on the penis and scrotum in men, on the vulva and perineum in women, and on the buttocks of homosexuals. The papules are symptomless unless secondarily infected and pustular, and the condition is sometimes only diagnosed when the patient attends because of some other sexually transmitted disease. The incubation period may vary from 3 weeks to 3 months, the lesions appearing individually or in crops, possibly due to auto-inoculation.

Management

When the condition is sexually transmitted the patient should be kept under serological surveillance for syphilis for 3 months from infection and all the known contacts examined. Treatment consists of destroying each individual lesion. This can be done by cryotherapy or by applying tincture of iodine or neat phenol on the tip of a sharpened orange stick into the centre of each lesion, taking care to protect the surrounding skin from the phenol if used. The treated papule will become white and a crust form before it heals. Further lesions may be found during the following 2 weeks and should be treated similarly.

PEDICULOSIS PUBIS

Pediculosis pubis is an infestation with *Phthirius pubis,* or the crab louse, of the pubic and peri-anal hair. While the infestation is usually confined to this area it can spread to the thighs, chest, axillae and eyebrows, but never to the scalp. It is almost always a sexually transmitted disease, but it can be acquired from infested bedding, towels or lavatory seats. The lice feed on blood and the chief symptoms is of an itch, which can be mild or severe, and which may not develop for several weeks after infection. With scratching the skin punctures may become secondarily infected. The adult lice are bluish-grey and pin-head sized. The hind legs, with which they attach themselves to the hairs have a span of 2 mm.

The female lays her eggs or nits at the bases of hairs. Each egg is contained in a chitin sac, cemented to a hair, and takes over a week to hatch. Lice have to be prised loose from the hairs with tweezers to be examined with a hand lens or with low power microscopy. The hair has to be removed for similar examination of a nit.

Management

All recent sexual contacts should be examined and the patient kept under serological surveillance for syphilis. Dicophane Application, B.P.C., is probably the most commonly used treatment. The emulsion is rubbed into the hairs of the pubis and surrounding areas, up to the level of the umbilicus, down to the knees, around the anus and any other area affected, and allowed to dry. One application should last about 3 days, but it is better to re-apply the emulsion on alternate nights, and whenever a bath has been taken, to allow a total treatment time of 10 to 14 days. This period is necessary as the chitin sac around the egg is impervious to dichophane (D.D.T.). Gamma Benzone Hexachloride Application, B.P.C., can also be used in a like manner. A single application of 0·5 per cent Malathion lotion appears to be equally effective as the eggs are also killed. Shaving the pubic hair is unnecessary, but some patients still feel 'itchy' after cure and are only relieved of their symptoms when they have shaved.

SCABIES

Scabies, or the itch, is a contagious disease due to infestation with *Sarcoptes scabiei.* The lesions of scabies are burrows in the skin, dug by the female acarus in which to lay her eggs. It can be transmitted asexually, as within families, by close bodily contact, or as a sexually transmitted disease. In the former case the distribution of the lesions is, in the finger webs, the ulnar borders of the wrists, the anterior axillary folds, the flanks, buttocks and genitals, in the latter it is predominantly on the genitalia. The irritation is most severe when the skin is warm, usually during the night, but rarely develops within a month of infection. Not infrequently scabies is found in association with other sexually transmitted diseases, sometimes the reason for the patient attending for examination.

The burrows appear as thin grey or black irregular lines on the top of elongated raised nodular lesions. On the shaft of the penis the nodules may be quite large. With scratching and secondary infection the burrows become long shallow ulcers. In men the lesions are commonly on the shaft of the penis, the prepuce or the scrotum, less frequently on the glans penis. They are more rarely found in women, mainly on the vulva. The diagnosis can usually be made clinically, but confirmation can be obtained by finding an acarus or some eggs in scrapings of a burrow which are mixed with liquor potassae on a glass slide and examined with low-power microscopy.

Management

All contacts should be examined: in the case of single people their sexual partners, but in addition the families of married patients. Serological tests for syphilis should be taken for 3 months from infection. Benzyl Benzoate Application B.P., is the most effective treatment for scabies. After an initial bath the emulsion is applied with a brush to the whole of the skin surface from the neck down and allowed to dry. This is done on three successive nights. On the fourth night the patient has a hot bath, the emulsion is scrubbed off and the underclothes changed.

Gamma Benzene Hexachloride Application, B.P.C. and Sulphur Ointment, B.P. are also effective. The single application of a lotion containing 1·0 per cent each of Dicophane B.P.C. and Gamma Benzene Hexachloride B.P.C. appears to be equally effective and this treatment can be carried out under supervision.

BALANO-POSTHITIS

Balanitis in the circumcised, and balano-posthitis in the uncircumcised have already been described as complications of gonorrhoea, trichomoniasis, candidosis and Reiter's disease, but these conditions account for only a minority of cases. Balano-posthitis is usually associated with a tight prepuce which, in some cases, cannot be retracted at all (phimosis) and the consequent lack of sub-preputial hygiene. The sub-preputial secretions (smegma) become infected, sometimes with anaerobic bacteria or Vincent's organisms which cause severe inflammation with tissue destruction. Because the anatomical defect persists, and even deteriorates, balano-posthitis tends to be relapsing and recurrent.

Symptoms nearly always follow two to three days after sexual intercourse. Initially the patient notices an irritation or soreness under the prepuce which is followed by preputial oedema together with a purulent and offensive sub-preputial discharge. On examination, when the prepuce can be retracted, a number of serpiginous erosions or ulcers will be seen on the inflamed and oedematous surfaces of the glans penis and the underside of the prepuce, especially in the coronal sulcus, the whole area being covered with a purulent exudate. When there is a phimosis due to inflammatory oedema or the scars from previous attacks, ulcers may be palpated through the prepuce and some peri-meatal ones seen on the inflamed glans penis. An associated inguinal adenitis, with tender and enlarged glands, is commonly found. Once the ulceration becomes established tissue destruction can be very severe indeed, especially if caused by anaerobic organisms. It is most important to exclude syphilis as the cause of the ulcers, by dark-ground examination of their secretions if obtainable, otherwise from sub-preputial saline washings. Only rarely is it necessary to do a gland puncture. Material for smears, wet films and cultures should be taken from the urethra and sub-preputial sac to identify the causal organisms. Operative procedures, such as circumcision, should be delayed until the inflammation has resolved; otherwise healing will be grossly delayed.

Management

Only rarely do the sexual contacts require examination, and then only when a specific cause has been found, but serological tests for syphilis should be carried out for 3 months from the last risk of infection. The initial treatment is with saline washes if the prepuce can be retracted, or by sub-preputial irrigations if not. The more frequent the treatment the quicker the cure. Patients with phimosis should be admitted to hospital, and if systemic treatment is required given a course of metronidazole or of a long-acting sulphonamide. Metronidazole, 200 mg thrice daily with meals for 7 days, or sulphamethoxypyridazine, 0·5 g twice daily for 5 days, is usually quite sufficient. In some cases, when syphilis has been eliminated, the phimosis may respond to alternate irrigation with a 1:4 solution of hydrogen peroxide and chlorinated soda surgical solution, B.P.C. Once the inflammation has resolved, circumcision can be performed which will rule out the possibility of further infections.

VULVITIS

Apart from the vulval irritation secondary to vaginitis due to trichomoniasis, candidosis and more rarely to gonorrhoea, or to vulval herpes, vulvitis is uncommon. It can be caused by lack of personal hygiene and contamination from the anus, the secondary infection of accumulations of smegma, the use of deodorant sprays which can cause local skin sensitivity, or the wearing of nylon underwear which is abrasive in the presence of moisture, whether due to perspiration or inflammatory discharges. Patients complain of irritation or soreness and a discharge. On examination there may be vulval excoriation, oedema and a discharge or only a mild inflammation.

Management

Whenever vulvitis follows sexual intercourse the consort should be examined and the patient kept on serological surveillance for syphilis for 3 months from infection. Treatment consists of personal hygiene, the daily washing of the external genitalia with a toilet soap and warm water, avoiding such irritants as deodorant sprays; the wearing of cotton underwear next to the skin will allow the absorption of perspiration.

PROCTITIS

Apart from gonorrhoea, candidosis, genital warts, primary and secondary syphilis which can all cause a proctitis, non-specific proctitis is rare. A number of passive homosexuals, and a very few women who admit to rectal intercourse, complain of rectal irritation of soreness and an anal discharge. On examination the rectal mucosa may be inflamed and covered in patches with a muco-purulent secretion. Only rarely does ulceration occur, with bleeding on palpation. Smears, wet films and cultures should be taken from the rectal lesions or secretions, in an attempt to identify the causal organism.

Management

If a cause is found then the contacts should be examined, the patient being kept on surveillance for 3 months from risk of infection. Most cases of non-specific proctitis respond to abstinence from intercourse and a course of sulphameth-oxypyridazine 0·5 g daily for 5 days, or of one of the tetracyclines, 250 mg six-hourly for 5 days.

PHIMOSIS

Phimosis is that condition in which the prepuce cannot be retracted over the glans penis. Normally the prepuce is freely retractable, but some degree of difficulty is experienced by a number of men and boys when the prepuce is too tight (partial phimosis) or even an inability to retract the prepuce if the opening is too small, congenital phimosis. Phimosis can also be acquired following attacks of balano-posthitis, when either adhesions form between the glans penis and the prepuce or the free margin of the prepuce becomes scarred, especially in the presence of glycosuria. Acquired phimosis almost always develops in the presence of an existing partial phimosis. Phimosis may cause difficulty in maintaining an erection and such pain that sexual intercourse becomes impossible. Occasionally it may cause difficulty in micturition, or even retention of urine. Normal sub-preputial hygiene is impossible and the secretions tend to become infected, causing repeated attacks of balano-posthitis. Middle-aged men with phimosis are at special risk of developing a carcinoma of the glans penis or prepuce, while any patient with a partial phimosis is liable to develop a paraphimosis during intercourse.

Management

It is rarely necessary to examine the sexual contacts of men suffering from phimosis except that their wives are said to be liable to develop carcinoma of the cervix, but patients should be kept on serological surveillance for 3 months from any risk of infection. The only treatment for phimosis, partial or complete, is circumcision. Many men with phimosis should have been operated upon when much younger, probably in infancy, and this would have saved them so much pain, discomfort and embarrassment. No phimosis improves, but with recurrent attacks of balano-posthitis gets steadily worse. Before operation the sub-preputial sac should be thoroughly irrigated to ensure that it is clean. Postoperative recovery is delayed if there is any infection at all.

PARAPHIMOSIS

Paraphimosis is the condition when a tight prepuce has been retracted over the glans penis but cannot be replaced. Oedema of the glans penis and prepuce follows, because the tight ring of tissue interferes with the blood supply and drainage. It only occurs when there is a partial or complete phimosis present to begin with. It is extremely painful and very embarrassing for the patient. On examination the prepuce is seen to be retracted proximal to the tight ring behind the glans penis, which may be discoloured, sometimes a plum colour.

Management

Serological surveillance should be carried out on the patient, but there is usually no necessity to examine the sexual contacts, unless the patient has some specific infection associated with the paraphimosis. Treatment is by reduction of the prepuce. Usually this can be done by firm but gentle compression of the oedematous prepuce and glans penis, taking plenty of time to reduce the swelling before slipping the constricting band over the glans penis. On occasions the band may need incision, under local anaesthesia, or the reduction have to be carried out under general anaesthetic. Once the inflammation has subsided the patient should be circumcised to prevent recurrence.

TRAUMA

Sexual intercourse is often associated with a certain amount of trauma. Usually the amount of discomfort experienced is insufficient to require medical aid, and the condition heals satisfactorily. Sometimes the damage is not noticed at the time, especially if the patient was drunk, but a number of men do develop bruises and abrasions one or two days later, usually on the glans penis or prepuce. With lack of cleanliness these often lead to balanitis or balano-posthitis. Similarly vulval and introital bruises or abrasions in women are liable to secondary infection, especially with enterobacteria, and cause vulvitis or vaginitis. In men more severe trauma can cause rupture of the fraenum or tears in the free margin of a phimotic prepuce, apart from a paraphimosis. There is immediate pain and bleeding, that from a torn fraenum possibly being persistent. Secondary infection is common unless the condition is treated early. In women the hymen may be torn at the first intercourse. Usually the bleeding is minimal, but on occasion can be severe enough to require haemostasis.

Chemical trauma of the genitalia usually follow attempts at self treatment with strong solutions of antiseptics or disinfectants, in an attempt at prophylaxis. Occasionally psychotics may use chemicals on their genitalia in attempts at self immolation. The results of the chemical trauma can vary from a dermatitis to burns or even necrotic ulceration, and they may mask an underlying sexually transmitted disease

Management

There is rarely, if ever, need for the sexual contacts to be examined, but the patient should be kept under surveillance if there has been any risk of infection. Most of the lesions due to physical trauma respond to simple hygiene. Excessive bleeding is usually controlled by compresses, but may need haemostatis of the bleeding points. Apart from hygiene, chemical trauma may require treatment with a bland and soothing application, such as boric acid lotion. Whenever secondary infection has complicated the traumatic lesion a course of sulphonamides should be given.

Psychotic patients who have injured themselves should be referred to a psychiatrist for treatment, initially as in-patients, as they are usually grossly disturbed mentally.

FURTHER READING

Callomon, F. T. & Wilson, J. F. (1956). *The Nonvenereal Diseases of the Genitals.* Sprinfield: Thomas.

Cobbold, R. S. C. & Macdonald, A. (1970). Molluscum contagiosum as a sexually transmitted disease. *Practitioner,* 204, 416.

Fisher, I. & Morton, R. S. (1970). *Phthirius pubis* infestation. *British Journal of Venereal Diseases,* **46,** 326.

Hutfield, D. C. (1970). Herpes genitalis as a venereal disease. *British Journal of Hospital Medicine,* **3,** 881.

Juel-Jensen, B. E. (1973). The chemotherapy of viral disease. *British Journal of Hospital Medicine,* **10,** 402.

Oriel, J. D. (1971). Natural history of genital warts. *British Journal of Venereal Diseases,* **47,** 1.

Teokharov, B. A. (1969). Non-gonococcal infections of the female genitalia. *British Journal of Venereal Diseases,* **45,** 334.

Wisdom, A. (1973). *A Colour Atlas of Venereology.* London: Wolfe Medical Books.

18. Other Conditions of the Genitalia

About a quarter of the patients who seek specialist advice do not, in fact, have any sexually transmitted disease. A number of men attend for check-ups, often without complaints, after a specific risk or before marriage, having run risks of infection in the past. Some patients have symptoms or lesions which they believe to be related to the genitalia, sometimes noticed following a specific risk, otherwise of either recent or long duration, but unrelated to any one risk, if indeed a risk has ever been taken. Their complaints may refer to:

(1) The normal architecture, or minor abnormalities, of the genital skin
(2) Pyogenic infections of the glands and follicles of the genitals
(3) Benign tumours of the genital skin
(4) Diseases of the genitals
(5) Premalignant conditions
(6) Malignant neoplasms
(7) Muco-cutaneous diseases with a distribution which includes, or is particular to the genitals
(8) Genital conditions associated with anxiety, neurosis or psychosis.

THE GENITAL SKIN AND ITS MINOR ABNORMALITIES

Many young men and adolescents notice, often after their first sexual intercourse, that the skin of the penis and scrotum differs from that elswhere. The prominent hair follicles and the rugae of the scrotum may appear to be a skin rash, and the median raphe a scar. Hirsuites papillaris are tiny swellings, or papillae, similar to early genital warts, which are scattered over the surface of the corona or the whole of the glans penis. In women the inner surfaces of the labia may have a granular appearance. The Fordyce syndrome consists of a harmless congenital defect of sebaceous glands, in which small white, or yellow, spots appear in the submucosa of the inner surfaces of the prepuce and the labia.

Firm translucent swellings may appear in the coronal sulcus following sexual intercourse or masturbation; these are lymphoceles and are caused by the temporary blockage of the lymph vessels. There is no treatment for these conditions. The fact that they are normal should be explained carefully to the patients who are usually anxious and often feel guilt. Reassurance is required. Varicosities of the veins of the scrotum cause varicocele, like a 'bag of worms'. They can be a cause of subfertility and may require surgical treatment.

PYOGENIC INFECTIONS

Infections with staphylococci and other pyogenic bacteria of the skin glands and hair follicles of the genitalia is not confined to the unwashed. Infections of the hair follicles on the penile shaft, scrotum, vulva or the pubic area, can cause acute folloculitis, chronic furunculosis or abscess formation, especially after misguided self treatment. Acute infections may follow others, such as pediculosis. Infections of the apocrine glands causes a hidroadenitis, usually in the axillae but also in the genito-anal region. The infection tends to be chronic and recurring. Tender, red swollen nodules slowly erode to the surface. Comedones can be seen in the glandular orifices. When infected, sebaceous glands become swollen, red and tender, later follicular cysts may develop. These retention cysts, usually seen in the scrotal or vulval skin as small yellow rounded swellings, may be hard or gritty on palpation, as the contents are prone to calcification. Chronic conditions of the sebaceous glands lead to acne.

Whenever there is a cause, such as pediculosis, it should be treated. Otherwise improved standards of hygiene, including washing twice daily with soap and water, and allowing perspiration to be absorbed, are all that is required. Rarely is systemic treatment required.

BENIGN TUMOURS

Benign tumours of the skin and subcutaneous tissues may affect the genitalia as elswhere. Fibromas usually affect the scrotum and labia majora. These firm painless swellings are sometimes pedunculated, and vary in size from a split-pea to a tennis ball. They have to be differentiated from the tender and grey-brown neurofibromas. Lipomas are soft or semifluctuant smooth masses with well-defined edges, which develop slowly on the vulva, mons pubis or the scrotum. Haemangiomas of all varieties may involve the genital region, including the mucosa, and be associated with similar lesions in the rectum and vagina. They are usually found on the shaft of the penis and scrotum in males, and on the labia majora and minora, the posterior fourchette and clitoris in females. Pigmented naevi (moles) of the genitalia are usually flat or slightly elevated and brown. In women the colour may deepen during pregnancy.

The treatment of pedunculated fibromas, if liable to trauma, is by removal. Lipomas need only be removed for cosmetic reasons. Superficial haemangiomas respond to cryosurgery, the deeper ones to sclerosis. Pigmented naevi should not be touched, unless increasing in size and suspected of being a melanoma, when a surgical opinion should be obtained.

ORO-GENITAL APHTHOSIS

Oral and genital erosions are found, together with ocular lesions, in two rare conditions of unknown aetiology: Stevens-Johnson's syndrome and Behçet's disease. The former is an acute, febrile and self-limiting condition with a very good prognosis, the latter chronic, relapsing and often with a fatal outcome.

Stevens-Johnson's syndrome

This condition is probably a clinical variant of erythema multiforme, and affects principally children and young adults. The onset is usually acute and with pyrexia. Aphthous ulcers or erosions develop on the mucosa of the mouth, tongue and fauces, the upper respiratory tract and occasionally of the lungs, causing a broncho-pneumonia. Similar lesions are found on the genital mucosa, those in the urethra causing a non-specific urethritis. The ocular lesions consist of an acute ulcero-membranous conjunctivitis, sometimes complicated by a keratitis. On occasions a nodular or vesicular eruption appears on the skin of the genitalia and the limbs. The erythrocyte sedementation rate (E.S.R.) is raised, there is a lymphocytosis and a bradycardia. Cultures from the lesions do not reveal any specific organism. The condition usually resolves within 2 to 3 weeks.

Stevens-Johnson's syndrome must be differentiated from Behçet's disease, Reiter's disease, syphilis, pemphigus vulgaris, foot and mouth disease and other causes of genital ulceration, which may be difficult when the disease is present in an incomplete form.

Treatment is mainly symptomatic; topical corticosteroids will relieve the pain and discomfort of the erosions and the eye lesions until recovery ensues. Secondary infection of the lesions, especially pulmonary, is the only danger, and should be prevented by adequate antibiotic cover, with penicillin or one of the tetracyclines. Systemic corticosteroids are rarely required, and then only for a short time.

Behçet's disease

Behçet's disease usually starts between the ages of 20 and 30 years, and is more common in men. Oral and genital erosions and a conjunctivitis may develop in any order. Relapses can occur after intervals of weeks or even years. The skin lesions vary from superficial painful herpetiform erosions to deep necrotic ulcers, each with an inflammatory halo, which heal with atrophic scars. In the male they are found on the scrotum, penis and inner thighs; in the female mainly on the labia majora. These latter lesions used to be known as 'acute vulval ulcers of Lipschütz'. In the mouth, pharynx and larynx lentil-sized mucosal erosions may develop into oozing ulcers. The ocular lesions may develop at any time up to ten years after the initial muco-cutaneous ones. The initial conjunctivitis may affect one or both eyes, and usually resolves in from 1 to 6 weeks, sometimes with impaired vision. The development of iritis, often with severe pain, is a dreaded complication as it is so often followed by hypopyon, leading to blindness.

Systemic complications are severe and include arthritis, effusions into the knee joints, thrombophlebitis and possibly multiple and diffuse lesions throughout the central nervous system, causing cerebellar, bulbar and brain stem damage as well as encephalitis or peripheral neuritis. Histological examination of the lesions shows evidence of a widespread vasculitis, with thrombosis and perivascular infiltrations of lymphocytes.

The differential diagnosis is as for Stevens-Johnson's syndrome. There is no known cure for Behçet's disease and treatment is symptomatic. The muco-cutaneous relapses of some women are associated with the menses; these may be suppressed by long-term oestrogen therapy. In general corticosteroids and the broad-spectrum antibiotics only give temporary relief, and then not consistently, but are always worth trying as may be immunosuppressive treatment with azathioprine.

BALANITIS XEROTICA OBLITERANS

This is a localized genital manifestation of lichen sclerosis et atrophicus. The aetiology is unknown and it can affect any age-group. The onset is usually insidious. A non-ulcerative atrophy of the skin and mucous membrane may affect the terminal urethra, the glans penis, the prepuce and, more rarely, the scrotum. Initially there is atrophy and depigmentation, followed by contractures which may cause meatal strictures or phimosis.

The patient may have noticed a mildly itchy white patch on the glans penis and, if around the meatus, difficulty in micturition, a thin stream of urine or, more rarely, retention of urine. If the prepuce has been affected he may complain of a phimosis. On examination white atrophic and contracted patches, sometimes surrounded with petechiae, are seen on a generally shiny glans penis. If the terminal urethra is affected the meatus will be firm and slit-like. Palpation of the terminal urethra may show that a sclerotic collar has extended 1 to 2 cm proximally. Preputial involvement causes progressive phimosis, white atrophic areas and fissures being found at the free margin.

In women a similar process involves the vulva, perineum and peri-anal areas, often in association with extragenital lesions. While most commonly seen in post-menopausal women, it can also develop in girls. The condition starts as white, irregular and flat plaques, which gradually become atrophic and shiny, sometimes pigmented at the periphery. Contractures of the vulval and introital lesions causes progressive irritation and dyspareunia.

The diagnosis is usually a clinical one but confirmation can be obtained by biopsy. There is acanthosis, thinning of the epidermis with subepithelial oedema, loss of elastic tissue, flattening of the papillae and lymphocytic infiltration. The treatment of phimosis is by circumcision. A cream containing hydrocortisone or fluocinolone acetonide, applied three times a day, relieves irritation and often causes the lesions to regress. A meatal stricture may be relieved by applying hydrocortisone ointment well into the meatus or, if more severe, by circum-meatal injections of hydrocortisone, in either case followed by regular dilatation with straight sounds for several weeks. Meatotomy is not advised.

PEYRONIE'S DISEASE

Peyronie's disease, or plastic induration of the penis, is a condition of unknown aetiology which usually affects middle-aged men. The initial complaint is of some pain in the shaft of the penis, worse during sexual intercourse, sometimes so severe as to preclude coitus. Later the penis becomes bent on erection, and this may make intercourse impossible. The cause of the complaints is a hard mass, or several masses, either nodules or plaques of a proliferation of sclerotic tissue which develops in, and dorsal to, the septum between the corpora cavernosa and must be differentiated from a malignant neoplasm. When removed at operation these masses resemble keloid tissue, and Peyronie's disease is often associated with Dupuytren's contracture.

On examination a sharply defined mass, or masses, firm as cartilage, can be palpated deep within the dorsum of the penis, the overlying skin being unaffected. The masses vary in shape from nodules, streaks and discs to that of a shield or saddle. The condition is very chronic and, while usually progressive, a number of lesions do resolve spontaneously.

Hydrocortisone acetate, 25 mg per ml, injected into the masses at weekly intervals for 8 to 10 weeks, is the most reliable form of treatment. Radiotherapy, with adequate shielding of the testes, is also effective in a proportion of cases. Surgical removal is only effective for small and solitary lesions. Oral treatment with vitamin E (100 mg thrice daily) or potassium p-aminobenzoate (12 g daily (24 tablets) in divided doses) do help a few patients, but the success of any form of treatment is difficult to assess because of the natural remissions which occur. Irrespective of the type of treatment relapse is quite common.

PRE-MALIGNANT CONDITIONS

There are two conditions of the genitals which, although not malignant, will undoubtedly become so in the course of time unless treated. Leucoplakia affects both men and women, while the erythroplasia of Queyrat mainly affects men.

Genital leucoplakia. Clinically and histologically genital leucoplakia resembles that of the oral mucosa and tongue. In men it is usually preceded by a chronic and relapsing balano-posthitis due to congenital phimosis, and in women by the menopause. Lesions on the glans penis and the under-surface of the prepuce in men, and on the vulva in women, appear as circumscribed, slightly elevated milky or bluish-white patches which become silvered and shiny. Erosions and ulcers may form and adhesions develop. Intense itching is common and can be very distressing. A clinical diagnosis should always be confirmed by biopsy.

Erythroplasia of Queyrat. The erythroplasia of Queyrat is a rare condition of unknown aetiology which usually affects the glans penis, only occasionally being found on the prepuce or the vulva. The lesions develop as circumscribed, flat, pink or red velvety patches which slowly increase in size, then remain unchanged unless, or until, they become malignant. The affected area is pliable, moist and shiny, but bleeds easily although ulceration is uncommon.

Histologically the appearances are of an intra-epidermal epithelioma, often indistinguishable from Bowen's disease, unless the rolled-up margins of the latter are seen. It is also similar to Paget's disease, although this is usually ulcerated. The diagnosis should always be confirmed by biopsy, the specimen being taken from the edge of the lesion.

Treatment

The treatment of pre-malignant conditions consists of destruction of the lesions by electrocautery or radiotherapy, circumcision being carried out in the case of preputial lesions. Whenever carcinomatous changes are present wide excision of the lesions, including partial amputation of the penis, should be done and followed by radiotherapy.

MALIGNANT DISEASE

Malignant neoplasms of the external genitalia are rare and most commonly develop after the age of forty. In men they almost always affect the uncircumcised, especially when the prepuce is phimotic, and there has been a recurrent and chronic balano-posthitis. In both sexes malignancy follows leucoplakia and the erythroplasia of Queyrat. Carcinoma may develop from chronic inflammatory lesions such as lupus vulgaris, from radiation burns, pigmented naevi or, more rarely, from benign tumours, e.g. angiomas and fibromas. In the past, epithelioma of the scrotum followed constant irritation with soot or coal dust; nowadays petroleum products are a more common cause. A basal cell epithelioma (rodent ulcer) is only exceptionally found on the external genitalia.

Bowen's disease. This is an intra-epithelial carcinoma which remains static for long periods, but in time will become a squamous cell carcinoma. The lesions are irregular, elevated and often red hyperkeratotic patches with rolled edges, the surface of which may become crusted or scaly. They may appear on the penis or the vulva, or at the anus.

Paget's disease. This is an intra-epidermal carcinoma which will slowly progress into a squamous cell carcinoma. The genital lesions are circumscribed, indurated raised nodules or plaques. Superficial ulceration takes place and the surface may be weeping or crusted, as in eczema.

Carcinoma of the penis. Carcinoma of the penis usually affects men over the age of 50 who have a partial or complete phimosis. It starts as a small scaly patch which becomes nodular or warty and rapidly ulcerates. In the early stages it is usually symptomless, but sub-preputial irritation or pain may occur. It can develop in several ways: as a firm infiltrating mass which invades the glans and the shaft of the penis, its surface granular and covered with a blood-stained purulent discharge; as an ulcerated infiltrative mass, the ulcers being raised and having rolled everted edges; as a fungating mass, with a foul smelling sub-preputial discharge and occasional haemorrhage, which may perforate through the prepuce. All these lesions may be palpable through the prepuce as hard tumours. At a late stage the inguinal lymph glands are involved, becoming enlarged and hard.

Carcinoma of the vulva. Carcinoma of the vulva is rare. It occurs mainly during the sixth and seventh decades, and most commonly affects the inner aspects of the labia, usually the majora, less frequently the clitoris. A nodule or wart develops on a plaque of leucoplakia and causes pruritus or soreness. The lesion develops into either an ulcer, with an infiltrated base, or a fungating warty growth. Vulval carcinoma metastasizes early and the inguinal lymph glands are soon involved.

Carcinoma of the cervix. Carcinoma of the cervix is the most common of genital carcinoma in women and occurs in the young and middle aged. Cervical *carcinoma-in-situ,* which can be cured by minor surgery, is being diagnosed with increasing frequency whenever routine cervical smears are taken for exfoliative cytology. It is found more often among women of the lower rather than the upper social classes, among the indiscriminately promiscuous, especially the longer they have been so, than those who are not, and among those with sexually transmitted diseases rather than those who have not. In women with antibody to type II *herpesvirus hominis* the condition appears to be more rapidly invasive than in those lacking antibody. It is rarely symptomatic, but an indurated ulcer may be seen on occasion adjacent to the cervical os. Haemorrhage, initially post-coital, may be an early sign.

Other genital carcinomas. Vaginal carcinoma is very rare. A warty growth or an indurated ulcer may be seen on the vaginal wall during a routine examination, or the patient may feel a lump.

SKIN CONDITIONS

A large number of patients who notice rashes or eruptions on the genitalia seek reassurance that the lesions are not sexually transmitted. The commonest symptom is irritation, which can vary from a mild itch to severe pruritus. Some of the skin conditions are infectious, others are generalized dermatoses or drug eruptions, although one of the commonest is neurodermatitis localized to the genito-anal region.

Herpes zoster. Herpes zoster or shingles is an infection caused by a virus identical with that causing chickenpox, but which affects the posterior spinal nerve roots. A segmental vesicular eruption develops within the sensory distribution of the affected root, or roots: in the case of the genitalia the third sacral root. A burning pain, possibly with an associated paraesthesia, is the initial symptom. This is followed by a patchy erythema, sometimes with fever, headache and malaise, and later by groups of large vesicles on one side of the penis and scrotum or the vulva, and of the perineum and one buttock. The vesicles become eroded, then either crusted or ulcerated. Secondary infection, with a painful inguinal adenitis, is common. Healing usually takes 2 to 3 weeks, leaving scars which are anaesthetic. A post-herpetic neuralgia may cause persistent pain over the distribution of the eruption.

Forty per cent idoxuridine in DMSO should be applied continuously for 4 days. Provided the patient is treated within a few days of the appearance of the eruption the chances of success are good. Infection can be controlled with sulphamethoxypyridazine 0·5 g daily for 5 days. Post-herpetic neuralgia often responds to hydroxocobalamin by injection, 1000 µg daily for 1 week.

Tinea cruris. Tinea cruris, or dhobie's itch, is a derma-tomycosis due to an epidermophyton which affects, and spreads from, the inguinal and genito-anal areas. The lesions are itchy, reddish patches with marginal papules and vesicles. The centre tends to heal, covered with minute crusts, as the lesion extends at the periphery. The condition is exacerbated by heat or moisture. A scrape from a lesion, mixed with liquor potassae on a slide, will reveal the mycelium. Local treatment is with Benzoic Acid Compound Ointment B.P.C. or Zinc Undecenoate Ointment B.P., but systemic treatment may be required to deal with resistant strains. Oral treatment is with Griseofulvin Tablets B.P. (500 mg), one being taken daily with the main meal for 6 weeks.

Erythrasma. Erythrasma may resemble tinea cruris or pityriasis versicolor in the genital region. The eruption is dark red-brown in colour with bright-red abrupt edges. The causal organism is *Corynebacterium minutissimum* and the diagnosis is best made with the use of Wood's light. Local treatment is with clotrimazole cream or one of the broad spectrum antibiotic ointments.

Seborrhoeic dermatitis. Seborrhoeic dermatitis rarely affects the genitalia alone; usually there are dry scaly patches on the scalp, spreading to the face, neck and trunk, together with dandruff. Itchy and reddish scaly lesions, with ill-defined edges, may be found on the penis and scrotum or the vulva, spreading to the inguinal and anal areas. Treatment in acute state is with 1·0 per cent hydrocortisone lotion, but when chronic with a 1·0 per cent sulphur and salicylic ointment.

Lichen planus. The violaceous lesions of lichen planus are usually found on the flexor surfaces of the wrists and arms, and just above the ankles. The cause of this usually chronic condition is unknown, but acute forms may be related to stress. On the vulva in women and the penis and scrotum in men the small polygonal flat-topped shiny papules may be arranged in annular fashion or scattered. The colour is purplish-red in dry areas and white in the moist, but all may be itchy. Often silvery lesions are also seen in the mouth, on the inner surfaces of the cheeks and on the tongue. There is no cure for lichen planus which usually disappears after a period of time and much more quickly after explanation and reassurance. When pruritus is severe it can be relieved with the application of 1·0 per cent hydrocortisone ointment.

Psoriasis. Psoriasis often affects the genitalia, but not as frequently as the elbows, knees and scalp. The cause is unknown, although there are probably genetic and psychogenic factors. In men the sub-preputial sac, the shaft of the penis and scrotum may be affected, in women usually only the vulva. The acute lesions are small bright red papules with silvery scales, but more commonly the lesions have become dull red or purplish plaques, and only covered with silvery scales in the dry areas. Some psoriatic patients develop an arthritis or have hyperkeratotic lesions on the soles of their feet, as in Reiter's disease. Psoriasis must be differentiated from a psoriasiform syphilide. There is no cure for psoriasis. Topical corticosteroids may help, but coal tar, in its various preparations remains the most effective treatment for this condition, whenever treatment is needed.

Contact dermatitis. Contact dermatitis is an acute eczematous dermatitis caused by allergens or by primary irritants. The former includes such allergens as poison ivy, transmitted to the genitalia by the hands. The external genitalia are liable to be affected by a number of irritants; in both sexes dyes in underwear, condoms, cervical caps, contraceptive creams and local medicaments, antiseptics, disinfectants, mercurial preparations and gentian violet; in women douches, pessaries, perfumes, deodorant sprays and sanitary towels with deodorizing chlorine-containing substances; in men cutting oils used in industry.

The pruritus can be controlled with local antihistamine preparations, sometimes supported by systemic drugs. The remedy is to avoid further contact with the offending agent, and this can only be discovered by careful history taking.

Fixed drug eruptions. The penis, scrotum and vulva are sites of predilection for fixed drug eruptions, which reappear at the same site whenever a drug is administered systemically. Usually these reactions consist of localized erythema and oedema with a vesicular eruption, but may simulate erythema multiforme, together with pruritus. Some drugs have a long history of causing these reactions in certain patients, antipyrin, phenolphthalein, pyramidon, phenacetin, salicylates and barbiturates. More recently some of the antibiotics have been incriminated, mainly penicillin but also streptomycin, chloramphenical and the tetracyclines. The most effective local treatment is with a corticosteroid such as 1 per cent hydrocortisone cream, but once again the cause must be identified and avoided by the patient.

Genital neurodermatitis. Pruritus of the genito-anal area, not due to any of the conditions already mentioned, is probably the most common of the non-sexually transmitted conditions of the external genitalia for which patients seek advice. In some cases the neurodermatitis may be due to allergy; in the majority the aetiology is unknown but, undoubtedly, anxiety plays a part whether the pruritus be predominantly genital or anal. It may be the presenting symptom of an underlying neurosis which requires psychiatric treatment. Occasionally there may be itching alone, but scratching and rubbing cause most of the objective findings, especially those of secondary infection. In acute cases the skin is oedematous and red, the surface oozing and crusted; when subacute there is less oedema, and a dull-red papular eruption can be seen on the dry and scaly skin; when chronic the skin may become lichenified.

The initial treatment is to control the pruritus with cortico-steroids and any infection with an antibiotic. Local applications usually suffice, such as an ointment containing 1 per cent hydrocortisone with 0·5 per cent kanamycin and amphomycin. In addition the patient should be instructed in personal hygiene, and, most importantly, the irritating factor, or factors, be removed. This may be as simple as anxiety or guilt after some sexual episode, but if it is more severe then the patient should be referred to a psychiatrist.

PRIAPISM

Priapism is the continued and painful erection of the penis, without sexual desire but with the ability to void urine. It is not associated with, or relieved by, ejaculation. Priapism is not common, but it can be caused by irritation of the nervi erigentes by diseases of the central nervous system or irritation of the peripheral nerves by pelvic inflammations. It can also be caused by restriction of the venous return from the corpora cavernosa, local trauma with thrombosis; conditions causing hyperviscosity of the blood, polycythaemia, sickle-cell anaemia; chemical intoxications, lead poisoning and aphrodisiacs; thrombophlebitis associated with acute prostatitis and seminal vesiculitis; carcinomatous or leukaemic infiltrations. In a few cases the aetiology remains unknown.

Aspiration and irrigation will relieve local stasis and thrombosis if followed by anticoagulants, which are used in the treatment of thrombophlebitis. Sedation and antibiotics should be used to treat inflammatory lesions, and palliative radiotherapy in those cases of malignancy.

PSYCHOGENIC COMPLAINTS

A number of patients seek advice because of apparent sexual dysfunctions. Some of these are physiological, nocturnal emissions and the loss of potency of ageing. Others may be due to anxieties, fears and justified feelings of guilt which can cause genital discomfort, impotence and frigidity, although they, and venereophobias may be the overt manifestations of more severe psychological disturbances including psychoses.

Nocturnal emissions. Adolescents and young men may become very anxious, and even neurotic, about occasional urethral discharges which occur during sleep. Rarely have they ever had sexual intercourse, and on examination are perfectly healthy. Nobody has explained to them that nocturnal emissions are physiological, that they happen to some frequently and others never, but that all are normal. Once the explanation has been given and accepted, the anxieties and neuroses disappear, and often the emissions as well. The same condition can occur in married men, especially if they tend towards neuroticism, when deprived of sexual intercourse for a time, as during a wife's illness or separation. Again the anxiety can be removed by explanation. On occasion a complaint about nocturnal emissions may mask anxieties about masturbation. Onanism is a normal phase in sexual development, and this should be explained, reassuring the patient that the only dangers of masturbation are the anxieties it may engender.

Genital discomforts. Some men complain of various vague pains and sensations in or around the genitalia. Some radiate down the groins or up the inner thighs, but all point, or terminate at the genitalia. On examination they are healthy. These symptoms are often the overt manifestations of anxieties and fears, not infrequently following promiscuous sexual intercourse. On occasion they may be caused by the worries and anxieties of everyday life and feelings of sexual inadequacy.

Reassurance is needed, and observation to exclude sexually transmitted diseases when the patient has been at risk. In some cases of severe neurosis the patients should be referred to a psychiatrist.

Impotence. Impotence is only rarely due to hormonal upsets or chromosomal disorders unless the man has never achieved an erection. Drug therapy can cause impotence, especially those used in the treatment of hypertension. The ganglion-blocking agents interfere with sympathetic and parasympathetic control and the sympathetic-blocking agents with ejaculation. Rauwolfia compounds may cause a depressive illness with an associated impotence. Centrally acting sedatives, especially the pheno-barbitones also depress libido. Impotence may follow trauma associated with sacral nerve damage such as fractures of the pelvis, and of the spine especially with paraplegia, although not all paraplegics are impotent. On rare occasions, impotence is caused by diseases of the central nervous system, tabes dorsalis and multiple sclerosis, or the neurological complications of pernicious anaemia and diabetes mellitus. In none of these is the prognosis good, despite intensive therapy. Certain operations, such as bilateral lumbar sympathectomy are followed by impotence, although with modern techniques that following prostatectomy is often psychogenic. Temporary impotence may occur in those debilitated after an illness, but when prolonged is almost invariably psychogenic. Most commonly it is an expression of depression, which may become deeper with the added anxieties of the impotence. Quite often recovery follows when this is explained to the patient, but in other cases counselling, with husband and wife together, is required before both will accept that he is normal. On occasion impotence is a manifes-tation of homosexuality, and as this may be latent, it is very difficult to treat. It is doubtful if a cure is possible, or even warranted. Impotence may be the presenting sign of an alcoholic, in which case control of the alcoholism will restore potency, although this may be delayed for several months if the alcoholism is of long standing. In other alcoholics impotence develops on their alcoholism being brought under control, the alcohol having been used to depress inhibitions. These patients, and in some cases drug addicts, will require psychotherapy before they can enjoy a normal sex life. In hypertensives, libido may return with a change in drug or an alteration in dosage, while treatment of the underlying depressive illness with chlorpromazine or one of the phenothiazines helps in those cases where that is the underlying cause of impotence. The use of mechanotherapy as an aid to supporting erection, has not yet been investigated sufficiently. It might have a place in the management of those with nerve damage but would appear to be of less help to those where the cause is psychogenic.

Frigidity. The term frigidity is usually applied to women who lack the ability to enjoy, and even have an abhorrence of, sexual intercourse. Such cases must be differentiated from those more common ones in which women have never, or only rarely, achieved an orgasm. In these cases, the cause usually lies in the poor techniques of the husband and may be remedied by its improvement. Sometimes it is found that the husband is impotent. The usual presenting symptom of frigidity is dyspareunia in the absence of a physical cause, such as vaginal or introital inflammation, maldevelopment or scars. The patients are very often depressed and the cause is almost always psychogenic. It may date back to past experiences, parental disharmonies or a sexual assault, or to a more recent episode such as the discovery of, or suspicion of, the husband's adultery, but much more commonly it is due to the fear of pregnancy. On rare occasions it is a manifestation of latent homosexuality. The psychological disturbance may either be a neurosis or a psychosis. The former will respond to explanation and reassurance, together with the provision of adequate contraceptive advice, on occasions the use of vaginal dilators but, of the greatest importance, needs the active co-operation of the husband or regular consort for success. Those with psychoses require psychotherapy, but the prognosis is not good.

Venereophobia. While a number of patients wisely seek reassurance that they have not acquired a sexually transmitted disease following a risk of infection, there are others who are convinced that they have such a disease, despite unequivocal evidence, from the specialist's point of view, that they have not. Some have run risks of infection in the distant past, others never (some not even having had sexual intercourse), but in all cases the clinical, bacteriological and serological findings are satisfactory. Despite explanations and reassurance from one specialist they will seek out another, and later, when he confirms the findings of the first one, yet others, sometimes returning to get more and newer tests done. The management of these patients is most difficult. One thing is certain: should they return without further risk of infection NO further tests should be taken. To do so can be taken by the patient as lack of confidence in the previous results, and therefore the current negative results can be questioned, with equal validity, at any future date. Whenever explanation and reassurance fail to convince such a patient, he or she, should be referred to a psychiatrist. Some obessionals respond to hypnotherapy, but a number are found to be psychotic, often schizophrenics, and in need of intensive psychotherapy.

FURTHER READING

Callomon, F. T. & Wilson, J. F. (1956). *The Nonvenereal Diseases of the Genitals.* Springfield, Illinois: Thomas.

De Costa, E. J. (1969). Infections of the vagina and vulva. *Clinical Obstetrics and Gynaecology,* **12**, 198.

Felstein, I. (1973). The organic causes of impotence. *British Journal of Sexual Medicine,* **1**, No. 2, 33.

King, A. & Nicol, C. (1969). *Venereal Diseases,* 2nd edn. London: Baillière, Tindall & Cassell.

Masterton, G. (1965). Oro-genital aphthosis. *British Journal of Venereal Diseases,* **41**, 292.

Percival, G. H. (1967). *An Introduction to Dermatology,* 13th edn. Edinburgh: Livingstone.

Willcox, R. R. (1964). *A Textbook of Venereal Diseases.* London: Heinemann.

Williams, J. L. & Thomas, G. G. (1968). Natural history of Peyronie's disease. *Proceedings of the Royal Society of Medicine,* **61**, 876.

Wisdom, A. (1973). *A Colour Atlas of Venereology.* London: Wolfe Medical Books.

19. Tropical Sexually Transmitted Diseases

The diseases, chancroid, lymphogranuloma venereum and granuloma inguinale, are found in the tropics and sub-tropics. Cases found in temperate climates are usually imported from abroad, but such is the speed and extent of intercontinental travel that cases may appear anywhere in the world. Their recognition in unexpected places is most important; otherwise local infections may occur.

CHANCROID

Chancroid, or 'soft sore', is a contagious disease typified by painful genital ulcers and suppuration of the inguinal lymph glands, an 'inflammatory bubo'. The condition is found occasionally in temperate climates when associated with lack of cleanliness. It used to be common among seamen, but no longer, now that shipboard hygiene has improved and treatment is available at sea. It remains very common in many tropical countries, in some areas being more prevalent than gonorrhoea. It is more commonly found in men than in women. The causal organism, *Haemophilus ducreyi*, was discovered by Ducrey in 1889. It is a short slender Gram-negative bacillus with rounded ends, and is usually found in chains or groups. The organisms are difficult to identify in pus from open lesions because of the large number of other bacteria present, but can be found in pus aspirated from an inguinal abscess. Culture is also difficult, special media being required.

Clinical manifestations

The incubation period is short, usually less than a week, and the initial lesions (solitary ones are uncommon), are almost always on the genitalia. The small painful and inflamed papules rapidly develop into pustules which break down to become sloughy based ulcers with undermined and ragged edges. Each ulcer is shallow, surrounded by a narrow bright-red zone, non-indurated and very tender. When the slough is removed the base is seen to be of very vascular granulation tissue which bleeds easily. The ulcers vary in size from a few millimetres to several centimetres, especially when several coalesce, sometimes in a linear fashion. Occasionally there may be marked tissue destruction, a phagedenic chancroid. In men the initial lesions develop in the sub-preputial sac, on the under-surface of the prepuce, the fraenum and the urethral meatus. In women they occur on the vestibule, the fourchette, the inner surfaces of the labia and the urethral meatus. Further lesions can develop from auto-inoculation on to the inner thighs and perineum, and in men on to the scrotum. The inguinal lymph glands, usually on one side, become tender, enlarged and matted together, forming a fluctuant unilocular abscess, bubo, of the groin. The skin over the abscess becomes red and hot, after which it almost invariably breaks down, a single sinus forming. The skin edges of the sinus may become chancroidal and a large ulcer develop which can extend to the thigh and the supra-pubic area.

Complications are localized to the genitalia and include phimosis or paraphimosis, urethral stricture, urethral fistula, severe haemorrhage and gangrene, especially if associated with Vincent's infection and phimosis. Although the incubation period is usually shorter, chancroid may coexist with early syphilis, lymphogranuloma venereum and granuloma inguinale.

Diagnosis

In practice the diagnosis of chancroid is usually made on clinical or therapeutic grounds, following the successful cure with sulphonamides, but not every tender genital ulcer is due to chanroid. Attempts should be made to identify *H. ducreyi* if not from ulcers, then from pus aspirated from an unruptured bubo. Smears are stained by Gram's method and cultures set up. The most commonly used culture medium contains defibrinated rabbit's blood, cystine, dextrose and beef-infusion agar. This is incubated at 28° to 32°C in a moist atmosphere for 48 hours. Biopsy from the edge of an ulcer may show certain microscopic characteristics; marked endothelial proliferation and palisading of the blood vessels, with thrombosis and infiltration of the deeper layers of the ulcer with plasma cells and lymphocytes. It is doubtful if the delay in starting treatment for this painful condition, while awaiting the results of the skin tests, is really warranted. The Ito-Reenstierna intradermal test comprises a suspension of killed *H. ducreyi* in normal saline. Dmelcos, a commercial preparation, contains 225 million organisms per ml: 0·1 ml is injected into the flexor surface of one forearm and an equal amount of normal saline into the other. A positive result is the development in 48 hours of an inflammatory papule, 5 to 10 mm in diameter, the control being normal. The test has its limitations; it does not become positive for 1 or 2 weeks after the initial lesions develop, and once positive, or after using Dmelcos, may remain so for life. A diagnosis can also be made by autoinoculation, as occasionally happens accidentally. Material from the edge of an ulcer is applied to a scarification on a normal area of skin, a similar lesion appearing within a week.

Management

Chancroid is often acquired in one place and treated in another. The source of the infection may be unknown, but all local contacts should be sought and examined.

It is doubtful if a chancroidal ulcer will respond to local hygiene alone, although many non-specific genital ulcers do. The sulphonamides are the drugs of choice in the treatment of chancroid. Streptomycin is equally satisfactory but its use may mask the early signs of granuloma inguinale. Penicillin is ineffective and, while the tetracyclines and chloramphenicol are effective, they may mask a developing syphilis, lymphogranuloma venereum and granuloma inguinale. Sulphadimidine or sulpha-diazine, 5 g daily in divided doses, are given for 10 to 14 days until healing is established. Sulphamethoxypyridazine, 1·5 g on the first day, then 0·5 g daily for 10 to 14 days is equally effective, but should not be given in late pregnancy. The dosage of streptomycin, when given, is 1·0 g daily, by deep intramuscular injection, for 7 days. When there is a secondary infection with Vincent's organisms metronidazole, 200 mg by mouth three times a day for 7 to 14 days, will aid healing.

The success of systemic therapy depends on maintaining drainage from all the lesions. Phimosis may require dorsal slitting of the prepuce, and later circumcision when the chancroid has healed. A fluctuant bubo may require repeated aspirations, always through healthy skin, to prevent sinus formation. Serological tests for syphilis should always be continued for three months from infection.

LYMPHOGRANULOMA VENEREUM

Lymphogranuloma venereum is a contagious sexually transmitted disease with a transitory primary lesion followed by suppurative lymphadenitis, and much later by serious local complications. It is much more frequently diagnosed in men than in women. The causal organism is a chlamydia, closely related to those which cause trachoma, inclusion conjunctivitis, oculogenital disease and psittacosis in man and enzootic abortion in ewes. The chlamydia, (formerly Bedsonia), are a group of organisms having similarities with viruses and bacteria, but more with the latter. The disease remains common in North and South America, the Caribbean Islands, West Africa, India, Malaysia and Southern China. It is also found in sea-ports throughout the world, although it is imported into temperate climates by travellers of all sorts, seamen, tourists and immigrants.

Clinical manifestations

The incubation period may vary from 1 to 6 weeks, but often is about 3 weeks. The primary lesion is a small transient, non-indurated, herpetiform lesion, in men on the glans penis, in the coronal sulcus or on the prepuce; in women on the vulva, the vagina or the cervix, the lymph drainage of the latter being to the pelvic lymph glands. Unless the lesion ulcerates and becomes painful the patient may not notice, or can ignore, it. Not all patients develop the more florid manifestations of the disease; some develop a temporary inguinal adenitis which resolves without suppuration or much pain, and a few men develop a chronic non-specific urethritis. Most commonly, however, the first complaint is of tender glands in the groin, usually unilateral, 1 to 6 weeks after the initial lesion. The onset of the inguinal adenitis is gradual, and in a few cases is accompanied by systemic upsets, fever, malaise, headaches and joint pains, even anorexia and sickness. Backache is more common in women and may be due to a pelvic lymphadenitis. Initially the glands are discrete, but with the peri-adenitis, they become matted and adherant to the skin and deeper tissues. The skin becomes bluish-red and a multiloculated abscess (bubo) forms which becomes fluctuant. Multiple sinuses develop, the discharging pus varying from caseous to blood-stained. Healing will occur eventually with scar formation, but sinuses may keep recurring. Women with initial lesions in the vulva or lower vagina develop an inguinal bubo as do men, but when it is in the vault of the vagina or on the cervix the pelvic and peri-rectal lymph glands suppurate. When the latter are affected the rectal wall becomes involved, causing an ulcerative proctitis, with a blood-stained purulent discharge. Passive homosexuals, with rectal lesions, develop a similar proctitis, and in both cases if they are not treated, may later develop chronic septic lesions, a peri-rectal abscess or rectal stricture, of which lymphogranuloma venereum is the only medical cause. Fistula-in-ano, recto-vesical or recto-vaginal fistulae and proctocolitis occur, with an associated chronic pelvic sepsis which alone may cause intestinal obstruction. In addition to suppuration of the lymph glands, the chronic inflammation of lymphogranuloma venereum causes a blockage of the lymphatics draining the genitalia, mainly in women, causing oedema and ulceration, and fistulae which open into the perineum, rectum and vagina. Vegetations and polyps may also appear on the perineum and around the anus. When the lymphatic oedema is gross it is termed elephantiasis or esthiomène. In women it affects the vulva, in men the penis and scrotum, and only rarely does the condition spread to the legs.

Diagnosis

The diagnosis is made on the clinical picture and the history of risk of an infection in an endemic area, confirmed by the results of the laboratory tests. Thin smears of pus can be fixed in methyl alcohol and stained with Giemsa's stain to identify Halberstaedter-Prowazek inclusion bodies, or fixed in acetone for fluorescent staining of the *Chlamydia*. Pus sent to the laboratory in Hank's medium or sucrose potassium glutamate can later be used for culture on BHK 21 or Hela cells. The Frei intradermal skin test uses as an antigen *Chlamydia*, grown in a yolk sac, and then killed. The commercial preparation is Lygranum, 0·1 ml of which is injected into the flexor surface of one forearm, an equal amount of the control material, prepared from uninfected yolk sac, into the other. The test is read at 48 hours, and when positive, an indurated red papule at least 6 mm in diameter will have formed at the test site, the control site being normal. Once positive, or following a Frei test, the reaction may remain positive for life.

The most sensitive serological tests for the diagnosis of

lymphogranuloma venereum are those recently introduced tests for *Chlamydia,* the radio-isotope precipitation (RIP) test and the micro-immunofluorescence (micro-IF) typing test. Either of these should be used, whenever available, in preference to the complement fixation test (LGVCFT) which is much less sensitive, but more so than the Frei test which is also less reliable. In the LGVCF test ovine abortion antigen, or one prepared from infected yolk sacs can be used. They are equally satisfactory, but only test for group antibody, strong positive results will also be obtained from those suffering, or who have suffered, from psittacosis and weak ones from those having trachoma or oculo-genital chlamydial disease. A titre of 1 in 16 or above is considered diagnostic in the presence of typical lesions. Much higher titres are commonly found in the early stages of the disease. Paired sera are not needed to diagnose lymphogranuloma venereum.

A rise in the level of immunoglobulins, especially of lgA, occurs early in the disease and is associated with an active infection. Observation of the immunoglublin levels is of importance when the LGVCFT has been found positive in the absence of other confirmatory findings. A normal lgA level would indicate a burnt-out or previously cured infection.

Management

Once the diagnosis has been established the patient should be interviewed about all possible sex contacts. Sulphonamides and tetracyclines are both effective in the treatment of lymphogranuloma venereum. Clinical improvement appears more rapid when the tetracyclines are successful, but there are cases in which the sulphonamides are more effective. Penicillin does not appear to be effective clinically. In the early stages treatment with one of the tetracyclines, 250 to 500 mg every 6 hours or doxycycline hydrochloride, 100 mg every 12 hours, either sulphadimidine or sulphadiazine, 5 g daily in divided doses for 14 days, is usually satisfactory. Once systemic therapy is established any suppurating bubos should be aspirated, and drainage encouraged from any sinuses and fistulae, by incision if necessary. In later lesions, especially in the presence of much scarring, the dosage of the systemic drugs can be doubled, the duration trebled and corticosteroids used to speed resolution. Prednisolone, 20 mg daily in divided doses for the first few days, then tailing off the dosage, may be of benefit. Surgery may be required after the initial course of systemic therapy, and should be carried out under antibiotic cover. Unresolved pelvic abscesses, often perirectal, may need drainage; intestinal obstructions and rectal strictures not responding to bouginage, will require excision and anastomosis. Elephantiasis may need treatment by a plastic surgeon. Surveillance of the early cases should be for 3 months when treated with sulphonamides and six when treated with tetracyclines.

There is, as yet, insufficient information available as to the time taken after treatment for the levels of the antibodies detected by the RIP and micro-IF tests to revert to normal. The titre of the LGVCF test usually falls quite rapidly after treatment, especially of early infection, and negative results may be obtained in 6 to 12 months, but in some cases the results remain positive for years. The levels of 1gA can also be monitored as a gauge to the effect of treatment and their reversion to normal used as a test of cure.

GRANULOMA INGUINALE

Granuloma inguinale is a chronic and usually sexually transmitted disease which remains common in parts of the tropics and subtropics. It is common in South America, the Caribbean Islands, India, Indonesia and the Pacific Islands; it is also found in West Africa, south China, northern Australia and the southern part of North America. It is rarely transmitted in temperate climates and is found in the Negro and coloured races. The causal organism is a Gram-negative bacillus with a distinctively large capsule when seen within mononuclear cells. It is now classified as *Calymmatobacterium granulomatis,* although it has long been known as *Donovania granulomatis,* or the 'Donovan body' after its discoverer. When stained with Giemsa's or Wright's stains the organisms appear as rods, with bipolar condensation of chromàtic material (like a safety-pin), lying within pink capsules. Electron microscopy studies have revealed cytoplasmic inclusions suggestive of bacteriophage. The incubation period usually varies from about 1 week to 1 month, but can be much longer.

Clinical manifestations

The initial lesion is a beefy-red painless papule or vesicle which ulcerates and slowly develops into a rounded and elevated velvety chronic granulomatous mass. It may appear on the genitalia, the groin, pubis, perineum or thighs, and in homosexuals at the anus or on the buttocks. The disease does not cause a lymphadenitis, but spreads by continuity and auto-inoculation as painless, friable, bright beefy-red ulcerative lesions. Progress is slow but the lesions can cover the genitalia, and in women involve the vagina, cervix and rectum. Healing is slow and is by scar formation, which often breaks down at a later date. Some ulcerative lesions become painful, especially when secondarily infected, as is common, sometimes with Vincent's organisms which cause phagedena, gross tissue destruction, offensive discharges and constitutional symptoms. Urethral stricture, cystitis, pyelitis and recto-vesical fistulae may develop. Obstruction of the lymphatics can cause gross genital oedema.

Diagnosis

The clinical diagnosis is made on the appearance of the beefy-red granulomatous lesions and the absence of lymphaden-itis. Confirmation is obtained by taking scrapings or biopsies from the edges of the lesions and making smears for staining by Giemsa's or Wright's method, screening the mononuclear cells for Donovan bodies, recognizable by their 'safety-pin' appearance. Biopsy material from the deeper layers of the ulcers may contain numerous plasma cells. In the early stages granuloma inguinale must be distinguished from condylomata lata, later the ulcerative lesions from epithelioma and lymphogranuloma venereum, also to be differentiated when there is lymphoedema.

Management

When the diagnosis is established the patient should be interviewed about all possible sex contacts. The tetracyclines and streptomycin are the drugs of choice in the treatment of granuloma inguinale, although erythromycin is also effective. Penicillin and the sulphonamides are not effective. Chloramphenical, which is, is not recommended for routine treatment because of its toxic effects. Tetracyclines are given in oral doses of 500 mg six-hourly or doxycycline hydrochloride 200 mg twelve-hourly for 10 to 15 days; streptomycin by deep intra-muscular injection, 1 g six-hourly for 5 days. Erythromycin can also be given by injection, 100 mg twice daily for seven days. Surveillance in early cases should be for 3 months when streptomycin has been used, and 6 months after the tetracyclines or erythromycin.

FURTHER READING

Davis, C. M. (1970). Granuloma inguinale. A clinical historical and ultra-structural study. *Journal of the American Medical Association*, **211**, 632.

Greenblatt, R. B. (1953). *Management of Chancroid, Granuloma Inguinale, Lymphogranuloma Venereum in General Practice.* U.S. Public Health Service Publication, No. 255.

Kerber, R. E., Rowe, C. E. & Gilbert, K. R. (1969). Treatment of chancroid. A comparison of tetracycline and sulfisoxazole. *Archives of Dermatology*, **100**, 604.

Lal, S. & Nicholas, C. (1970). Epidemiological and clinical features in 165 cases of granuloma inguinale. *British Journal of Venereal Diseases*, **46**, 461.

Manson's Tropical Medicine (1960). 15th edn, edited by P. H. Manson-Bahr. London: Cassell.

Rajam, R. V. & Rangiah, P. N. (1954). *Donovaniasis.* World Health Organization Monograph Series, No. 20.

Schacter, J., Smith, D. E., Dawson, C. R., Anderson, W. R., Deller, J. J., Hoke, A. W., Smartt, W. H. & Meyer, K. F. (1969). Lymphogranuloma venereum–I. Comparison of the Frei test, complement-fixation test and isolation of the agent. *Journal of Infectious Diseases*, **120**, 372.

Wisdom, A. (1973). *A Colour Atlas of Venereology.* London: Wolfe Medical Books.

20. The Tropical Treponematoses and Endemic Syphilis

The tropical treponematoses, yaws and pinta, are contagious diseases caused by treponemes indistinguishable from *T. pallidum* microscopically, although there are sub-microscopic differences. Bejel and endemic syphilis are similar diseases, probably caused by *T. pallidum,* while endemic syphilis has occurred in temperate climates as well as in the tropics. All these diseases run a milder course than does sexually transmitted syphilis, from which they also differ epidemiologically. The origin of these various diseases, and, of course, of syphilis, is unknown. Some believe that they have all arisen from a single source; that they have adapted themselves to survive the various environmental factors found in different parts of the world, and that the individuality of clinical manifestations are those which give the best chance of spread under the different circumstances. On the other hand, sexually transmitted syphilis, yaws and the other treponematoses may be found in neighbouring areas, and at one time in Scotland, syphilis

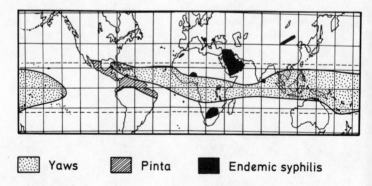

░ Yaws   ▨ Pinta   ■ Endemic syphilis

Fig. 12 Distribution of tropical treponematoses and endemic syphilis.

existed in two forms, one endemic (sibbens), the other sexually transmitted.

The World Health Organization has undertaken mass treatment campaigns in various parts of the world, in an attempt to eradicate the prevalent treponematosis by testing whole populations, or as many as were available, and treating all those infected. Of the various campaigns in Thailand, Indonesia, Nigeria, certain Caribbean Islands and Yugoslavia, only the last seems to have eradicated the treponematosis from the population.

YAWS

Yaws is a chronic contagious disease found in those parts of the world where, at least for part of the year, there is high humidity and tropical heat. The causal organism, *Treponema pertenue*, is indistinguishable microscopically from *T. pallidum*. Infection with yaws does give some immunity against infection with syphilis. Transmission is usually by close bodily contact in infancy or childhood, but spread may be by insect vectors or via fomites, while a few are congenital, or rather neonatal, from mother to foetus. It is common in certain Caribbean Islands, in parts of South America, in tropical Africa, Ceylon, Malaysia, Thailand, Indonesia, northern Australia and the Pacific Islands. It is rare in the Indian subcontinent and China.

Yaws is divided into three stages, primary, secondary and tertiary, although lesions of two stages often coexist. Histologically the early lesions, primary and secondary, are characterized by oedema, polymorphonuclear leucocyte and plasma cell infiltration of the skin and an interpapillary invasion of the corium by the epidermis. *Treponema pertenue* are found in the cellular infiltrations. The tertiary lesions are gummatous, necrotic and ulcerative, with much granulation and scar tissue formation. The perivascular infiltration and endothelial proliferation is less marked than in syphilis, although they may be indistinguishable microscopically.

Clinical manifestations

Primary yaws. The incubation period is usually about 4 weeks, a primary lesion developing at the point of entry. This is usually on the leg, but may be in the mouth of an infant. A single painless, but possibly itchy, papule or ulcer develops into a crusted granuloma, rather like a raspberry, and called a fram-

boesioma. *Treponema pertenue* and blood exude from the surface
when the crust is removed. The lesions vary in size from 1 to
5 cm. On the sole of the foot it may be painful, and is called a
'crab-yaw' because of the gait adopted. The regional lymph glands
become enlarged and constitutional upsets, malaise, headaches and
nocturnal bone pains may occur. Untreated the lesions heal in a
few weeks, unless secondarily infected, in which case healing may
be delayed for months. The serological tests for syphilis, reagin
tests, RPCFT, TPHA and FTA-ABS, usually become positive
about 3 or 4 weeks after the appearance of the primary lesion,
the TPI test taking somewhat longer.

Secondary yaws. The secondary lesions appear about 1 month
after the primary but may be delayed up to 3 months. They
consist of generalized papular or papillomatous eruptions, which
come in crops over a period of 2 years, sometimes associated with
constitutional symptoms. A generalized enlargement of lymph
glands is usual. Individual lesions start as yellow papules which
coalesce with neighbouring ones. The surface of the hypertrophic
lesion thus formed becomes eroded and granular, with pink raised
areas which soon become covered with a crust from the dried
serous exudate. These lesions are referred to as framboesiae. Most
of the lesions in the secondary stage are on limbs, few are on the
trunk. Their configuration may vary widely, some form plaques,
others are annular or serpiginous. The skin in between active
lesions may become hyperpigmented. On occasions the skin is not
broken and the lesions are nodular. In moist areas the lesions tend
to be condylomatous; on the palms and soles they are often
hyperkeratotic, on the soles sometimes ulcerated and painful, i.e.
'crab-yaws'. Papular lesions commonly appear on the mucous
membranes, especially of the mouth, independently of those on
the skin. Healing of the secondary lesions is with scarring and
changes in pigmentation.

Bones may be affected by an osteitis, with areas of rarefaction,
or a periostitis of the long bones, with the deposition of
sub-periosteal new bone, a 'sabre-tibia' being quite common.
Polydactylitis affecting both fingers and toes is also common.
Juxta-articular nodes or ganglia may appear at the wrists. Painless
effusions into the knee joints may also occur. Hypertrophic
osteo-periostitis of the maxilla causes the development of a bony
tumour called 'goundou'. This is usually found in children
following a rhinitis, with a purulent discharge, like 'snuffles'. The

tumour can develop to such an extent as to obstruct vision, and even destroy the eye by involvement of the orbit, the facial skin remaining unaffected throughout. Relapses of secondary lesions may occur at varying intervals up to 5 years from infection, and may affect the skin, mucous membranes or bones.

Late yaws. The late, or tertiary, lesions may develop within a year of the early ones healing, or may follow after several years of latency. Most of the lesions are gummatous and heal with tissue loss and scarring. In the skin, superficial or deep ulcers heal with 'tissue-paper' scars and surrounding hyperpigmentation some-times with contractures. Large areas of the skin may become thickened and depigmented; the palms and soles are often fissured and eroded, causing severe hyperkeratosis. Bone lesions are very common, the skull being affected frequently. Dactylitis of the proximal phalanges may cause a shortened digit if a phalanx is destroyed; gummatous osteitis with necrosis can cause pathological fractures, or extend to the surface with ulceration. Perforation of the palate and nasal septum is caused by a painful ulcerative process, 'gangosa'. It is associated with a foul-smelling purulent discharge and an especially offensive halitosis. The cardiovascular and central nervous systems are not affected in yaws, which rarely has fatal lesions. Nevertheless, the debility it produces so weakens patients that they succumb to intercurrent infections which they would otherwise survive.

Diagnosis

The diagnosis should not be difficult in those areas where yaws is endemic. The lesions are quite characteristic and *T. pertenue* can be demonstrated in serum from the early skin and mucosal lesions when examined by dark-ground microscopy. All the serological tests for syphilis become positive within a few weeks of the primary sore, and remain so even when the disease has become inactive, although the reagin tests may become negative.

In temperate climates active late yaws may be present in a very few cases but the diagnosis may be difficult, or even impossible in some cases when the condition is latent. The diagnosis may be made from the history, or the finding of 'stigmata' of previous lesions. The patient may remember having had injections in childhood for 'bad blood' or during a World Health Organization mass campaign. Careful clinical examination may reveal the stigmata: areas of depigmented skin, 'tissue paper' scars on the legs, hyperkeratosis on the soles of the feet, spindle thickening of the phalanges, and X-ray evidence of periostitis of the long bones, especially of the tibiae. The reagin tests are usually positive, but only at a low titre, the cardiolipin Wassermann reaction often being negative.

Treatment

Penicillin is the drug of choice in the treatment of yaws. Active yaws usually responds to one injection of from 1·2 to 2·4 mega units of procaine penicillin in oil with aluminium mono-sterate (P.A.M.), as used in the mass campaigns of the World Health Organization. Late or latent yaws, when diagnosed in a temperate climate is usually treated as for latent syphilis, namely 600 mg (1 mega unit) of procaine penicillin by injection daily for 10 days.

PINTA

Pinta is a relatively mild and chronic contagious disease with a good prognosis, which is endemic, and in certain areas epidemic, in Mexico, Central America and northern South America. It has also been reported in some Caribbean and Pacific islands. The causal organism, *Treponema carateum,* is indistinguishable micro-scopically from *T. pallidum,* but cross-immunity between pinta and syphilis is not certain. The serological tests become positive as in syphilis and yaws. Transmission is by skin contact in childhood, there being no evidence of congenital infection. The lesions are divided into primary, secondary and tertiary stages. Histologically the lesions are characterized by thickening of the epidermis, which may contain an excess, or absence, of melano-phores, together with the infiltration of lymphocytes and plasma cells into the perivascular spaces and the dermis. *Treponema carateum* are present in secretions from the early lesions.

Clinical manifestations

The incubation period varies from weeks to months, the primary lesion appearing on the legs, arms or face. The initial lesion is a papule which spreads to become a psoriasiform, reddish, scaly patch, or 'pintid', later surrounded by similar papules. *Treponema carateum* are present in the serous exudate. The regional lymph glands become enlarged. Several months later the secondary stage develops with a generalized indolent eruption of papular or squamous patches, 'pintids', which tend to coalesce. They vary in colour from pink to deep violet, and are scaly. Hyperkeratosis of the soles and palms is common. All the secondary lesions are very chronic, and may last for years.

The tertiary stage is characterized by pigmentary changes. Initially there is an increase of pigment on the hands, wrists and legs where the raised, dry and scurfy patches may become dull red or slate blue, and sometimes itch. Later the lesions become atrophic and depigmented, leading to widespread leucoderma, which is so unsightly as to cause great distress to the unsophisticated patients. Cardiovascular and neurological complications do not occur.

Diagnosis

The diagnosis is based on the clinical findings in a patient with a rural upbringing in an area where pinta is endemic. Many lesions are psoriasiform, but *T. carateum* are present in the early lesions, and the serological tests are usually positive well before secondary stage, but not as early as in syphilis or yaws.

Treatment

Pinta has been treated successfully in the mass campaigns with a single injection of 1·2 mega units of PAM.

BEJEL

Bejel is a chronic treponemal disease which affects about 60 per cent of the members of the nomadic tribes of Bedouins who move about the Euphrates valley, Syria, Iraq and the Arabian peninsula. It is probably a form of endemic syphilis and its transmission, in an environment of squalor, filth and primitive, overcrowded living conditions, is by bodily contact, eating and drinking utensils, and possibly by insect vectors.

Clinical manifestations

The majority of infections occur in childhood. The first noticeable lesion is a mucous patch on the site of an angular stomatitis due to avitaminosis, or within the mouth, further lesions appearing in the mouth and throat, sometimes causing hoarseness, and at the anus, where they often become condylomatous. The generalized skin eruption may be papular or squamous, and is often either annular or erosive. There is usually a generalized enlargement of the lymph glands. Periosititis and osteitis, with nocturnal bone pains, are found, but constitutional symptoms are uncommon and mild. Treponemes, probably *T. pallidum,* are present in serum obtained from early lesions which heal within 2 years, leaving the patient with latent bejel. In some tribes over 90 per cent have serological evidence of treponematosis. The tertiary stage may take years to develop and the lesions are mainly gummatous. Those of the skin heal with dipigmented scars, alopecia and a fissured hyperkeratosis of the soles. Osteitis and periostitis occur in the long bones, but a gummatous condition of the nasal bones may produce disfigurement. Many lesions become secondarily infected which may cause constitutional symptoms and even chronic ill health. Congenital infection does not occur, nor are the cardiovascular and central nervous systems affected.

Diagnosis

The diagnosis is made on clinical grounds, but treponemes are present in the early lesions and the serological tests for syphilis are positive in all established cases.

Treatment

The World Health Organization mass campaign in Iraq obtained satisfactory results with a single injection of 1·2 mega units of PAM, the dose being repeated within a week when bony lesions were present.

ENDEMIC SYPHILIS

The non-sexual transmission of syphilis can occur in communities living in primitive and overcrowded conditions typified by abysmal lack of hygiene. In the past, endemic syphilis was known in Scotland as sibbens, in Ireland as button-scurvy and in Scandinavia as radesyge. More recently it was present in the Bosnia area of Yugoslavia, the Borgas area of Bulgaria and in the Inner Mongolian Republic of the USSR. Currently it exists in Botswana (dichuchwa), Rhodesia (njovara), South Africa, Northern Nigeria and Southern Morocco, while a small outbreak has been reported from Vienna. Transmission is probably by commonly used eating and drinking utensils.

Clinical manifestations

The disease is common in infants and children. The initial lesion is usually found on, or around, the mouth. The manifestations appear to be identical to those of bejel. Occasional cases of congenital infection are recorded, but they are rare because infection of girls is usually at a very early age.

Diagnosis

The diagnosis is made on the clinical findings, together with the detection of *T. pallidum* in the early lesions, and the finding of positive serological tests for syphilis.

Treatment

In the very successful World Health Organization mass campaign in Yugoslavia, a single injection of 4·8 mega units of PAM was used.

FURTHER READING

Batchellor, R. C. L. & Murrell, M. (1961). *A Short Manual of Venereal Diseases and Treponematosis,* 2nd edn. Edinburgh: Livingstone.

Du Toit, J. A. (1969). Endemic syphilis in the Karoo. *South African Medical Journal,* 43, 355.

Expert Committee on Venereal Infections and Treponematoses. Fifth Report (1960). World Health Organization Technical Report Series, No. 190.

Grin, E. I. & Guthe, T. (1973). Evaluation of a previous mass campaign against endemic syphilis in Bosnia and Herzegovina. *British Journal of Venereal Diseases,* 49, 1.

Guthe, T. (1969). Clinical serological and epidemiological features of framboesia tropica (yaws) and its control in rural communities. *Acta dermato-venereologica, Stockholm,* 49, 343.

Guthe, T. & Idsøe, O. (1968). The rise and fall of the treponematoses—II. Endemic treponematoses of childhood. *British Journal of Venereal Diseases,* 44, 35.

Hudson, E. H. (1957). *Non-Venereal Syphilis.* Edinburgh: Livingstone.

Luger, A. (1972). Non-venereally transmitted 'endemic' syphilis in Vienna. *British Journal of Venereal Diseases,* 48, 356.

Manson-Bahr, P. H., editor (1960). *Manson's Tropical Diseases,* 15th edn. London: Cassell.

Morton, R. S. (1967). The sibbens of Scotland. *Medical History,* 11, 374.

Simons, R. D. G. Ph. & Marshall, J., editors (1969). *Essays on Tropical Dermatology.* Amsterdam: Excerpta Medica Foundation.

Wisdom, A. (1973). *A Colour Atlas of Venereology.* London: Wolfe Medical Books.

21. Tropical Diseases Affecting the Genitalia

The time is long past when doctors could afford to be parochial about the conditions they had to diagnose. Such is the speed of travel today that diseases contracted within a week, but half the world away, may have to be diagnosed and treated. Each year there is an increasing amount of intercontinental travel, which is reflected in the rising numbers of patients being seen with 'exotic' conditions. Some of the travellers are immigrants, others the employees of oil companies, civil engineering contractors in developing countries, working as fitters or technicians, apart from students, business men, members of the armed services and their families, air-crews, and the largest group of all—tourists. Merchant seamen rarely travel by air in any numbers, but when abroad often do come in contact with the native populace. A number of diseases, usually confined to the tropics and subtropics, may have genital manifestations which can cause the sufferers to fear that they have acquired a sexually transmitted disease. Exceptionally, some of these diseases, when they can be transmitted by close bodily contact, are passed on during sexual intercourse.

VESICAL AND RENAL CALCULI

Urinary calculi are one of the most common conditions encountered in the tropics. The vesical ones are much more frequent and affect especially boys and young men. Little is known about the cause, but a highly concentrated urine associated with sweating, and a diet lacking sufficient vitamin A, have been suggested. It is very common in south China. In Africa, where urinary schistosomiasis is prevalent, eggs of *Shistosoma haematobium* often form the nuclei of urinary calculi.

Clinically the patients may present with a persistent non-specific urethritis, haematuria or dysuria due to the passing of 'gravel'. The urine often becomes secondarily infected, and there may be a history of renal colic. Acute retention of urine may develop, temporary or intermittent when a stone falls over the internal urethral meatus, but permanent, until relieved, when a stone blocks the posterior urethra.

The diagnosis is made by cystoscopy or by X-ray examination of the urinary tract, and treatment is carried out by a genito-urinary surgeon.

TUBERCULOSIS

Tuberculosis is now rare in Britian and many of the developed countries, but in other parts of the world it remains prevalent, and is associated with urban squalor.

Primary tuberculosis lesions may appear on the penis, scrotum or vulva, infection being by contagion. A nodular or pustular lesion appears about 1 week after infection and becomes ulcerated. The ulcer is tender, yellowish-red, with serrated and undermined edges and an associated inguinal adenitis. It must be differentiated from a chancre.

Late tuberculous lesions of the genitalia are either varieties of lupus vulgaris or of scrofuloderma. The former affects the penis, scrotum or vulva with irregular ulcers, serpiginous scaly lesions or a hypertrophic form with chronic oedema; scrofuloderma of the inguinal and genital regions follows an inguinal adenitis, with ceseation, abscesses or indolent sinuses which leave radiating scars.

The diagnosis is made by finding *Mycobacterium tuberculosis* in the early leasions and by biopsy of the later ones. Further investigations and treatment should be undertaken by a specialist in tuberculosis.

CUTANEOUS DIPHTHERIA

Diphtheria is rare in the tropics, but is found in the subtropics as a disease of civilization in the towns and centres of population. Skin lesions are found in South Africa (veld sore) and in the Middle East and North Africa (desert sore). Occasionally genital lesions are found in the sub-preputial sac and on the vulva. The initial lesion is a painful vesicle filled with straw coloured fluid which develops into a tender shallow ulcer. It becomes chronic in 2 to 3 weeks, punched out and circular, with an undermined edge and thickened margins; on the vulva a widespread swelling develops which is firmly indurated and reddened. The base of the ulcer is covered with grey scaly debris, underneath which is an adherent membrane. These may take over a year or more to heal.

The diagnosis is made by isolating *Corynebacterium diph-*

theriae from the primary lesion and treatment is with anti-diphtheritic serum.

LEPROSY

Leprosy is found throughout the tropics, and to a lesser extent in the subtropics, while occasional cases and even 'pockets' are found in temperate climates, although it is essentially a disease of rural communities. The incubation period is long, usually 1 to 2 years, but may be as long as 8.

The commonest genital lesion is an orchitis which causes testicular atrophy and may result in sterility, sometimes with gynaecomastia. Nodular lesions, occasionally found on the penis, scrotum and vulva, vary in size from one half to several centimetres in diameter. Yellow-brown or brown-red skin infiltrations are also found; they vary in shape and consistency, and may simulate a chancre. There is usually some disturbance of sensation, either anaesthesia or paraesthesia.

Leprosy is diagnosed by identifying *Mycobacterium leprae* in smears made from scrape-incisions of the lesions. A proportion of patients have false-positive reactions to the reagin tests, the specific ones being negative unless the patient is also suffering from a treponematosis. Treatment with the anti-leprotic drugs is best left to the experts.

FILARIASIS

A number of nematode worms, which live in the lymphatics and connective tissues, produce live embryos, which enter the blood stream, and cause lesions in the urinary tract and on the external genitals.

Wuchereria bancrofti

The distribution is throughout the tropics and subtropics; it is very common in India and southern China, but extends to the southern parts of the USA, southern and eastern Europe and Australia. The mosquito is the intermediate host. The incubation period is at least 3 months. Blockage of the lymph vessels by the worms and invasion of the tissues by the larvae may cause abscesses, sometimes in the scrotum, lymphangitis, with varicosities of the inguinal lymph glands, or a lymphoedema of the scrotum, or vulva, which may progress to elephantiasis. Orchitis, funiculitis, hydrocele and chyluria, sometimes blood-stained, may also occur. The milky chylous urine will coagulate if left standing.

Night blood is taken for the diagnosis of the microfilaria, but the condition can also be diagnosed by a specific complement fixation test and intradermal test.

Loa loa (loaiasis)

Loaiasis is found between the Congo delta and Lake Victoria. The intermediate host is the mangrove fly. The incubation period varies from 1 to 3 years. Transient subcutaneous swellings, Calabar swellings, measuring 2 to 3 cm across and painless but hot, appear and disappear within 3 days. A hydrocele or a localized abscess of the groin may develop on the death of a parent worm. Severe pain occurs when a loa wanders into the urethra.

The diagnosis can be made either by finding microfilariae in the blood, by use of the specific complement fixation test or by an intradermal test.

Onchocerca volvulus

Human onchocerciasis is found throughout the whole of central Africa and in Central America. The intermediate host is the jinja-fly or one similar.

Subcutaneous tumours, 0·5 to 5 cm in diameter, may be painful, often at 15 day intervals. Genital lesions include lymphatic enlargement of the scrotum, hydrocele with an enlarged testis, elephantiasis of the scrotum and 'hanging-scrotum', skin containing sclerosed enlarged femoral or inguinal lymph glands.

The diagnosis is made by finding *Onchocercae* in skin biopsies made near a nodule.

Dracunculus medinensis (Guinea-worm)

Dracontiasis is found in the Nile valley and as far south as Uganda, in West Africa, Arabia, Iran and in parts of Brazil. The intermediate host is a freshwater crustacean, a cyclops, which is ingested in drinking water. The female worm appears on the skin, usually of the feet, about a year later to discharge her eggs.

Very occasionally, when a worm dies, it can cause a scrotal swelling with urticaria, or even an abscess.

The diagnosis is usually made clinically, but X-rays may show calcified worms in the tissues.

CUTANEOUS LEISHMANIASIS

Leishmaniasis in the form of oriental sores is found in northern Nigeria, along the Mediterranian littoral and the Middle East, as well as in Central Asia, the west coast of India, China and South East Asia. It is also found in Central and South America. In the tropics it is commonly seen at the beginning of the cold season, and in more temperate climates in early autumn. The intermediate host is the sandfly and the incubation period varies from days to weeks, or even months.

The causal organism, *Leishmania tropica,* is a parasite of the reticulo-endothelial system, and lesions usually appear on the uncovered parts of the body, but occasionally they are found in the perineum and peri-anal region. On the vulva, and in the vagina, they are sexually transmitted. A minute itching papule expands as a shotty infiltration of the dermis, becoming covered with fine scales. A crusted shallow ulcer forms which spreads peripherally, leaving a central horny spicule 2 to 3 cm in diameter, or even longer. Some papules do not ulcerate, but develop as scaly and scabbed flattened plaques which are to be distinguished from chancres.

The diagnosis is based on the clinical findings, and confirmed by the presence of Leishman-Donovan bodies in the aspirates taken from beneath an ulcer, or by an intradermal test.

GENITO-URINARY SCHISTOSOMIASIS

Bilharziasis is found throughout Africa, the Middle East, South America and the Caribbean Islands. The intermediate host is a freshwater snail, excretion from humans being mainly in the urine. The incubation period varies from 3 months to 2½ years.

The vast majority of patients have no complaints. The commonest symptom is terminal haematuria, with or without dysuria. Sometimes clots are passed. On occasion, a milky urethral discharge is present in which eggs may be found by microscopic examination. The pain may be dull and suprapubic, or acute, with frequency and urgency. When rectal ulcers are present, blood and mucus will be passed in the stools. The haematuria may last for months or years, and then resolve unless the patient is reinfected. In severe cases cystitis may supervene, often with secondary infection, and vesical calculi develop around the eggs. Prostatitis and seminal vesiculitis may cause sperma-torrhoaea, involvement of the ureters and kidneys may result in hydronephrosis. Bladder papillomas develop in some cases. Because of the persistence of the haematuria the patient becomes severely anaemic and debilitated, and a prey to intercurrent infections.

In men infiltration by the eggs causes urinary fistulae opening into the perineum or the posterior surface of the scrotum; urethral strictures, which are fairly common; epididymitis and funiculitis. Women may suffer from peri-urethral abscesses, scarring of the Fallopian tubes and ovaries, with subsequent sterility; papillomatous lesions of the urethra; inflammation of the vagina, cervix, vulva, anus or the groins.

The diagnosis is made by finding the eggs in the terminal urine, by biopsy of the bladder, or by a specific complement fixation test during the first 3 years of the disease, and by an intradermal test.

AMOEBIASIS

Amoebiasis is found throughout the tropics and subtropics, while sporadic outbreaks occur in the temperate climates. The incubation period varies from 1 week to 3 months.

The causal organism, *Entamoeba histolytica,* is a cause of dysentery but diarrhoea is not invariable in amoebiasis. Cutaneous involvement is secondary to that of the bowel, by contamination with infected stools. The peri-anal and perineal areas are affected most commonly, the spread being facilitated by excoriation. The glans penis and the urethra may be involved in homosexuals. An amoebic granuloma may spread over a wide area, causing firm infiltrations, warty growths and a vegetating necrotic ulceration which, in women may spread to the vulva and vagina.

The diagnosis is made by finding the *Entamoeba histolytica* in scrapings from early skin lesions or, using a proctoscope, from the rectal walls.

FURTHER READING

Callomon, F. T. & Wilson, J. F. (1956). *The Nonvenereal Diseases of The Genitals.* Springfield, Illinois: Thomas.

Carruthers, R. K. & Long, S. V. (1970). Genito-urinary tuberculosis in an area with a large Asian immigrant population. *British Journal of Urology,* **42**, 535.

Manson-Bahr, P. H., editor (1960). *Manson's Tropical Disease,* 15th edn. London: Cassell.

Simons, R. D. G. Ph. & Marshall, J., editors (1969). *Essays on Tropical Dermatology.* Amsterdam: Excerpta Medica Foundation.

Symposium on Imported Disease (1970). *Transactions of the Royal Society of Tropical Medicine,* **64,** 199–238.

Index

Printed by T & A Constable Ltd., Edinburgh

NOTES